COMMUNITY MEDICINE

A Study Guide

Heinemann Medical
Student Reviews

Community Medicine
A Study Guide

Professor ROY D WEIR
OBE MD (Aberd) DPH FRCP FFCM
Head of Department of Community Medicine
University of Aberdeen

GEORGE INNES
MD (Aberd) DPH MRC Psych FFCM
Reader, Department of Community Medicine
University of Aberdeen

ELIZABETH M RUSSELL
MD (Glas) Dip Soc Med DObst RCOG FFCM MRCP (Glas)
Senior Lecturer, Department of Community Medicine
University of Aberdeen

Heinemann Medical Books
London

Heinemann Medical Books,
22 Bedford Square,
London WC1B 3HH

ISBN 0–433–35000–8

First published 1988

British Library Cataloguing-in-Publication Data

Weir, Roy D.
  Community medicine: a study guide.
  —(Heinemann medical student review).
  1. Community health services 2.   Public health
  I. Title   II. Innes, George
  III. Russell, Elizabeth
  362.1′0425   RA425

  ISBN 0–433–35000–8

Typeset by Wilmaset, Birkenhead, Wirral and
printed in Great Britain by Biddles Ltd, Guildford

Contents

Contents

Preface

THE GUIDE TO STUDY

In Aberdeen the original stimulus for a study guide was a reduction in whole class teaching, a move to tutorials and the need to find an economic means of presenting previous lecture material. The aim was not to produce a textbook but, as the title implies, a guide for individual student study. The material, intentionally, requires to be supplemented by tutorial and personal work either as set essays or problem-based projects. It is, however, flexible and the main sections may be done in any order allowing different tutors in different years to contribute to the course and providing the necessary background, at any stage, for a variety of projects.

The purpose of the *Guide* therefore is to pull together a single, compact yet readable account of the different elements in a community medicine course. The individual sections of the further reading lists are other authors' versions of these same topics. None is intended as a primer to be memorized; the aim is to provide a number of descriptions from which the student's understanding will grow. It is not intended as a detailed account of community medicine but rather an *index and guide* to the items *that should be studied by students during a community medicine course.*

As it is seldom possible to deal in detail with all the course material during lectures or small group teaching, it is assumed that students will complement those formal contributions by working systematically on their own using the *Guide* and further reading lists at the end of each section. The *Guide* is divided into four main sections with a

short introduction which describes the concerns and activities of
community medicine and a final chapter suggesting priorities for
research.

COURSE CHECK LIST

The overall aims of the course are to introduce undergraduates to the
human context of clinical method and science. The bulk of the course
is therefore intended to provide knowledge which students will apply
in clinical practice.

In general terms students who complete the course should:

(1) be aware of the need for a method of scientific evaluation in
    medicine and of the general principles of such evaluation
(2) be able to handle numerical data about groups and calculate
    various rates
(3) know the sources of information related to health and be able to
    answer analytical questions on such data
(4) be aware of the effects of behaviour on health and disease,
    prevention and treatment
(5) be familiar with the relative effectiveness of medical care versus
    other non-clinical intervention in changing the course of common
    diseases
(6) be aware of the nature and operation of health services.

More detailed aims are given at the beginning of each section.

Contributors

Maria Bergmann, MB (Berlin), MFCM
Mildred L Blaxter, MA (Oxon. Aberd), PhD
David R Cohen, B Com (McG), M Phil
George Innes, MD (Aberd), DPH, MRC Psych, FFCM
Gavin H Mooney, MA (Edin)
Elizabeth M Russell, MD (Glas), Dip Soc Med, D Obst RCOG,
    FFCM, MRCP (Glas)
Roy D Weir, OBE, MD (Aberd), DPH, FRCP, FFCM Head of
    Department

Chapter

1

Introduction to Community Medicine

EVOLUTION OF CARE ● CHANGES IN MEDICINE ● MISCONCEPTIONS
OF 'NEED', 'DEMAND' AND 'EFFECTIVENESS'

The purpose of this chapter is to describe the concept of community medicine. It shows the origins of the techniques outlined in later chapters of the Guide and describes briefly how and why these techniques are used by community medicine specialists in looking at the health problems of groups of people rather than of individuals and how the web of natural history and causation is explored. This approach, formalized in the practice of epidemiology, first ascertains and describes the distribution and determinants of disease in man and thereafter seeks to promote the health of human communities. The goal, of course, is to investigate cause and thereby initiate prevention. Examples of successful ventures can be found in *Uses of Epidemiology* (Morris, 1975).

EVOLUTION OF CARE

In looking at health and the health service today, it is worth recalling how the various services evolved in the UK.

The first phase was concerned with the care of the *destitute*. Historically this was an enormous problem and attempts to deal with it started in the 1600s with the Poor Laws which were variable, unequal and often unfair. The process was slow, even harsh, but ultimately led to a national system which is the basis of our present social security. In 1834 the Poor Law Act attempted to remove the subsidizing of low wages and, indeed, the whole object of this phase was to achieve a basic level of subsistence.

Obviously the phases overlapped and the next, the period of *sanitary reform*, was precipitated by a huge problem, if not a crisis. In the first half of the nineteenth century, the population of Great Britain doubled from 9 to 18 million; it also shifted into the towns, and the wealthy as well as the poor were found to be susceptible to the diseases of the day. The cholera outbreaks of 1831 and 1853 and the 25 000 annual deaths from smallpox in the 1880s are obvious examples. In 1870 a whole series of acts was introduced to clean up and improve the material environment.

In the third phase after 1870, concern shifted from the environment to personal health. The first major development in *health care* came with Lloyd George's National Health Insurance Act of 1911 which set out to provide medical care for employed men with an income below a certain level. The scheme established the concept of a panel of patients – the beginning of general practice as we know it today.

The penultimate phase centred on 1948 with the advent of the *National Health Service*. This period was stimulated by the depression of the 1930s and the whole wave of social reconstruction following two world wars. The health service was, of course, only one part of a much larger system and only one act of a whole legislative series attempting to deal with sickness, unemployment, education, housing and social security which originated from the Beveridge Report (1942).

It is inevitable that these evolutionary phases will continue and the next one is concerned with achieving both a proper *balance between medical and social services* and a reorganization of their financing. As a consequence, the need to determine the individual's and the state's responsibility in health and health care is now more clearly recognized.

It is still possible today to see all these various phases in the components of the present system into which they have evolved. Care for the destitute was the forerunner of social security and sanitary reform established the present system of environmental control. Such control need not be detailed here but neither should it be taken for granted. The need for adequate amounts of safe water and appropriate methods of waste disposal are as critical now as they have ever been, although the control and responsibility is no longer medical. These problems vary the world over – some areas have no clean water supplies and no sewage disposal. In developed countries the problem is quantity – more and more water is being demanded and greater amounts of waste (not just sewage) have to be disposed of; details of the resulting health problems and the appropriate forms of control are given in later sections.

CHANGES IN MEDICINE

As diseases change, so must services adapt. Medical services must keep in step with changes both in medicine and in society; community medicine's concern is with the effect of this interaction. For example in the last 50 years there have been five major trends in society:

(1) the composition of society has changed, with more elderly and fewer young people
(2) social differences in education and job opportunities have narrowed
(3) living standards have risen and, with these improvements, dietary and other habits have changed
(4) the expectations of individual members of society have increased
(5) society is increasingly dependent on technology.

In medicine, as a result, there are corresponding changes:

(1) a different mix of diseases has resulted from the changes in the population and in society
(2) a shortage of health workers has arisen because of more attractive careers elsewhere
(3) increasing technology has concentrated resources in hospitals
(4) both social and technical changes have required health service staff to work as members of teams
(5) the speed of change is such that accepted methods of practice are likely to alter at least twice more during our professional working lives.

Ironically, despite all the changes in medical practice, the expanded ability to treat illness and the increase in resources, there has been no major change in death rates, except in those under the age of 25 and, more particularly, in the infant mortality rate throughout the period since the health service was established. This raises the question of whether the services and developments over this period have been wholly appropriate or whether mortality is no longer the best measure of effectiveness.

The problem is that there is no reliable measure of morbidity (i.e. illness or disability), let alone health. The really disturbing feature is the difficulty in obtaining information about the extent to which the different kinds of care and treatment required by the population at different times are provided and, when provided, with what result. We know a good deal about what services are used, but it is essential to distinguish 'use' from 'need' and 'demand'. To improve health the basic activities in community medicine are directed towards three aims:

(1) to help people make sound choices about health and health care
(2) to determine the medical services needed (rather than demanded)
(3) to find out if the services which are provided meet these needs.

MISCONCEPTIONS OF 'NEED', 'DEMAND' AND 'EFFECTIVENESS'

The concepts of 'need', 'demand' and effectiveness are frequently misunderstood.

Need refers to those people who have a problem which medical care might help whether or not they ask for it.

Demand is generated by those people who seek help whether or not they actually have a medical 'need'.

Effectiveness refers to the efficacy of services in meeting 'need' and combines the concepts of whether treatment actually improves the outcome and whether services as a whole are aimed at the most important medical problems.

The ways of defining need and subsequent effectiveness in meeting needs are major topics for discussion. This is a very real issue because the health service is under pressure and there is a danger that we may seem to do what is technically possible in part because it *is* possible, without making a real assessment not only of the amount of need for that service, but also of the resulting benefit compared with other problems. Unfortunately, it is all too seldom that such comparisons are made when health priorities are determined. This latter point raises the issue of resources and costs and, even if more money were made available for health care, choices would still have to be made because of our ability to do so much more.

When the National Health Service started it was believed, because of our experience with infections, that disease could be contained – it was not anticipated that by saving the lives of the young they would then survive to develop the diseases of ageing and thus again require the input of health resources. Indeed, our very expensive technical advances save the lives of people who, though surviving, may then be completely dependent on medical and social services and so further raise expenditure.

The questions we must keep asking are:

(1) *What are our health problems and what services do we provide?*
First define the health problems facing the population: what are they, how many people are affected and what is being done about them? Next, look for the most appropriate method of dealing with them: by prevention; by screening and early detection; by long-term surveillance and by home or hospital care.

(2) *Do our services solve our problems, what sort of services should we provide?*
Measure the success with which the above problems have been solved. Would we be better off with new types of staff and completely new types of services? Having defined the problems, their size, our success and the alternative solutions, our next step is to provide more appropriate services – training or retraining staff, modifying or developing existing services. Finally, the cycle is started again by measuring the success rate.

These are the issues and tasks with which community medicine is concerned and it is against this background that this book should be viewed. Attention is focused on the questions of who in the community needs care, could these needs have been prevented, what sort of care is required and, when provided, is it effective?

Understanding of these problems is based on four major topics:

(1) methods of investigation: epidemiology; economics; information services; evaluation (Chapter 2)
(2) prevention including occupational health, environmental control and the basic practices upon which health is built (Chapter 3)
(3) the provision of medical and social care: how to recognize and accommodate the need for change and ensure effective care (Chapter 4)
(4) health and behaviour: how to work with people and help the community to take a fresh responsibility for its health (Chapter 5).

From these presentations an indication is given of *how* the problems ought to be tackled. A further aim is to show *why* such questions must be asked. An examination of the past shows that at different points of time particular problems stand out which had to be overcome. A hundred years ago the problems were environmental and the need for sanitary reform offered both a challenge and a solution. Fifty years ago the therapeutic explosion changed the problems to those of ensuring that new and complex technical treatments were effective and safe.

Today, in the face of these advances, the problems are how to provide and organize access to this care. In the past there was perhaps too little that could be done for most patients, now there is almost too much for at least some conditions. As a result and to avoid inappropriate and uneven use, the need today is to learn how to choose well, who to treat, and in what way. Everyone makes such choices every day but may be unaware of them. As in the past, the challenges to doctors and other health workers are to be able to ask questions, recognize solutions and, above all, adapt to change. The speed of change in society around us is increasing and the success of medical care in future depends on its ability to keep pace with and accommodate these changes.

REFERENCES

HMSO (1942) *Social Insurance and Allied Services*. London: HMSO (Sir William Beveridge Report, Cmnd. 6404)

Morris, J. (1975) Four cheers for prevention. In: *Uses of Epidemiology*. Edinburgh: Churchill Livingstone

Chapter

2

Methods of Investigation

DEFINITIONS AND TECHNIQUES USED IN EPIDEMIOLOGY • HEALTH
ECONOMICS • INFORMATION SERVICES • AN EVALUATIVE
FRAMEWORK • MAIN SOURCES OF HEALTH CARE INFORMATION •
NOTIFIABLE DISEASES • ASSESSING THE 'HEALTH' OF A
COMMUNITY • INTERNATIONAL VARIATIONS IN DISEASE

To assist in answering questions about identifying our health
problems and the extent to which our health service meets these
problems, community medicine uses various methods and measurements. These are described in this chapter.

OBJECTIVES

Students should know:

(1) the epidemiological method of studying disease causation
(2) the main sources of information about disease and death in the UK
and how the data are collated from individual to national statistics
(3) at least in general terms, the epidemiology of:
(a) the more common cancers (e.g. lung, alimentary, urogenital,
haemopoietic)
(b) the major cardiovascular diseases (e.g. coronary artery disease,
hypertension and stroke)
(c) other chronic degenerative and occupational disorders (e.g.
chronic bronchitis, arthritis, pneumoconiosis and asbestosis)
(d) significant infections and tropical diseases (e.g. rubella,
whooping cough, malaria)
(4) for these more important medical conditions, the size of the
problem – morbidity and mortality; the relationship to age, sex,
occupation, personal habits and living conditions; time trends and
geographical variations; and current hypotheses of causation and
the evidence for them.

Students should be able to:

(1) apply the epidemiological method of analysis to their clinical knowledge of a disease
(2) interpret data and assess the validity and generalization of conclusions of an epidemiological study
(3) calculate simple incidence and prevalence rates
(4) list, for any individual, the factors known to create risk of particular diseases and outcomes
(5) design an investigation of an epidemic of an acute or chronic disease
(6) recognize the continuing application of epidemiology in day-to-day clinical practice.

Students should appreciate:

(1) the philosophy of evaluation and the need to know that the treatment they give is effective, acceptable and making the best use of resources
(2) the concept underlying the process of peer review (or medical audit) and the need to participate in such exercises.

DEFINITIONS AND TECHNIQUES USED IN EPIDEMIOLOGY

Epidemiology is the study of the distribution of disease in man and the factors determining that distribution. Its purpose is to understand how and where disease arises, leading ultimately to the prevention of that disease. Although it is the main investigative technique of community medicine, it is of relevance to all those who work with objective methods in clinical practice and research. The basic approach is to apply systematic or mathematical techniques to problem solving.

The epidemiological method

In the past, one of the most obvious ways in which a health problem was recognized and measured was its association with death. There were two reasons why this came about. First, death was a very definite outcome, with the event and associated illnesses frequently recorded, initially in church records and later nationally through official registration. Second, death gave an indication of the seriousness of the disease. It was noted that diseases were not randomly distributed throughout a population, but rather that each followed a pattern, affecting certain groups or individuals more than others. Epidemiology is concerned with the *extent* and *types* of illnesses in various groups of people and with the factors that influence their distribution. Over the years the concepts and practice of epidemiology have been ordered into definable stages which overlap to some extent, but all start with items of information and suspicion which are then systematically analysed to try to produce evidence of associations or causes of ill-health.

Recognition

The first essential is to recognize either that a new problem has appeared or that an existing problem seems to have a particular pattern. This may sound self-evident, even superfluous, but it requires an alertness to changes in the type of patients or problems which present themselves in surgery or clinic and a willingness to question previously held assumptions. There are good reasons why recognition of new disorders or associations may be slow. A single doctor seldom sees a sufficient number of patients for any change to be detected unless it is very sudden or serious. The realization that even minute variations in the amounts of the active ingredients in contraceptive pills were associated with heart disease was delayed because of the fact that hundreds of thousands of women had for many years been taking 'the pill' apparently safely. The evidence, however, had been there all the time and it only required that the right question be asked.

Usually, the awareness starts with a comment to colleagues (Fig. 2.1) and grows haphazardly at first until there is enough of a suspicion to move to the next stage, the beginning of systematic enquiry.

Definition

After raising the suspicion, there is the associated task of agreeing and defining the condition that is being studied, i.e. *from what* is the patient suffering: symptoms, signs and as exact a diagnosis as possible including, where appropriate, the results of laboratory investigation. In an individual patient the evidence justifying clinical action is seldom complete. To insist on defining precisely what is wrong before treating a patient would cause unacceptable delay in clinical practice, but in

Is Thalidomide to blame?

SIR, — I feel that four cases which have occurred in my practice recently are worthy of mention, as they may correspond to the experience of other practitioners. They all presented in more or less the same way—each patient complaining of: (1) Marked paraesthesia affecting first the feet and subsequently the hands. (2) Coldness of the extremities and marked pallor of the toes and fingers on exposure to even moderately cold conditions. (3) Occasional slight ataxia. (4) Nocturnal cramp in the leg muscles. Clinical examination in each case has been essentially negative, and during this time I have not noticed similar cases in my practice.

It seemed to me to be significant that each patient had been receiving thalidomide ("distaval") in a dose of 100 mg. at night, the period during which the drug had been given varying from eighteen months to over two years. Thalidomide is generally regarded as being remarkably free of toxic effects, but in this instance the drug was stopped. Three of the patients have now received no thalidomide for two to three months, and there has been a marked improvement in their symptoms, but they are still present. The fourth patient stopped taking the drugs two weeks ago, and it is therefore too early to assess the effect of withdrawal.

It would appear that these symptoms could possibly be a toxic effect of thalidomide. I have seen no record of similar effects with this drug, and I feel it would be of interest to learn whether any of your readers have observed these effects after long-term treatment with the drug. I might add that I have found it otherwise to be a most effective hypnotic with no "morning hang-over" effect. It has been especially useful in patients with skin pruritus and discomfort.—I am, etc.,

Turriff, Aberdeenshire.   A. LESLIE FLORENCE.

Figure 2.1 Recognizing a problem (from *Br. Med. J.*, 1960, Dec. 31).

population surveys such definitions are essential. As a result much effort in epidemiology has gone into clarifying diagnostic labels and into rigorous standardization of diagnostic methods. This apparently double standard is justified because of the different purposes and effects of treating an individual patient compared with an entire population.

Ascertainment

Next comes the stage of 'ascertainment', i.e. finding and counting all the people with the defined condition. Although reliable records will give a picture of all patients seeking medical advice for a specified disease, special surveys may be required to show the range of severity of the condition and the proportion of sufferers from that disease who seek medical advice. This aids the clinician by giving a more precise picture of the prognostic significance of specific signs and symptoms than does a study of a hospital group or of known patients alone. The importance of such population-based surveys was exemplified in studies of sudden death, in which the results revealed the size and unrecognized urgency of the problem of cardiovascular deaths outside hospital. To this end the routine recording of cases so that their relative frequency in different groups can be compared is a fundamental task of community medicine.

Association

The prime aim of ascertaining the number of cases is to seek the causes of disease by noting and analysing its frequency according to variables such as time or season, geography or the habits and characteristics of those affected by it. Such analysis shows how those with the disease differ from those who are not suffering from it. *When* did this happen: which year, season, even time of day; the periodicity of outbreaks. *Where* did this happen: country, town, specific focus of disease in school or factory; geography; geology; meteorology and sociology. *To whom* did this happen: what attributes are common to all those affected; genetic, anatomical, physiological, serological, occupational. In addition, an apparent association *between* diseases is worth exploring because, if confirmed, it may point to a common cause or to a common pathogenic mechanism. Thus the study of associations suggests *hypotheses* about causes of disease. Before putting such hypotheses to the test, it is essential to consider whether they are biologically plausible. The sale of margarine from the 1940s to the 1970s increased in line with the increase in lung cancer, but there is no biological basis for suggesting that margarine causes cancer. On the other hand, it was biologically plausible to hypothesize a causal relationship with the increase in sales of cigarettes, hence the subsequent intensive search for proof of a *direct* or causal association.

Verification

Hypotheses on causation suggested by the patterns of mortality and morbidity must be put to the test of controlled comparisons of the experience of both sick and well. It is important to have a close and continuing link between the broad look at routine data such as national death rates and the intensive study of matched groups of patients and appropriate controls. Thus, although the cause of death on death certificates is known to be often inaccurate, pointers to possible causes may be found in national tables of mortality which show links with factors such as age, sex and occupation. The recognition of deaths in young asthma sufferers due to the overuse of aerosol inhalers is a good example. On the other hand, the more recent technique of long-term natural history studies has the advantage that they start with apparently well people whose habits and characteristics can be ascertained by observers unbiased by any knowledge of their subsequent fate. Other types of study used to verify hypotheses are described below.

Application

After verification there is the application of the knowledge gained, sometimes the most difficult step of all. Here the aims are either primary prevention, whereby the disorder is avoided, or detection at a stage when some reversal is still possible. Experience of large or migratory populations living in different circumstances points to the importance of certain adverse effects on those studied. For example, incipient lung disease is found in children exposed to air pollution and cigarette smoking. Although the lesson for medicine must be that to change environment or habits may be by far the most potent method of either prevention or cure, there are considerable difficulties in achieving such changes which are discussed in Chapter 3. Broadly, primary preventive action may be taken at three different levels of society:

National action: Parliament enacts that we must or must not do something, with a penalty for non-compliance. An example is the Clean Air Act, 1956, which forbids the emission of dark smoke everywhere in the UK. This act was passed when it was shown that smoke pollution of the atmosphere contributed to the development of bronchitis and, under certain atmospheric conditions, to smog formation with many resultant deaths in the young and old.

Local action: a local authority which decides to fluoridate its water supply is taking minority social action as a result of epidemiological investigations into the hypothesis that the addition of one part of fluoride to one million parts of water reduces the prevalence of dental caries in children.

Voluntary action (individual or group): when an individual gives up smoking because of the finding that it is associated with the development of cancers of the lung and bladder and of coronary artery disease, he or she is part of a widespread but uncoordinated action by society.

These types of social action may all be occurring at the same time and with the same end in view.

The *role of epidemiology* in medicine is changing; not only has the context of its application shifted from acute infections to chronic diseases of uncertain origin, but the concepts and practice of the discipline are now being applied to health problems as well as to diseases. Examples are the monitoring and improvement of prescribing practices and the detection of iatrogenic disorders and adverse reactions. Similar methods are applied to the supervision and organization of long-term care of patients with thyroid disease and other chronic disorders, the aim being to monitor and detect early any complications of the disease or its treatment. Thus a cycle or feedback loop is established by regular recording, and the treatment is thereby continually being refined. When aetiological enquiries lead to the consideration of methods of primary prevention or early detection, as in screening for cancer, rigorous and, more important, statistical methods are used in the planning and analysis of the controlled trial of such procedures to test and monitor their efficiency. For example, this is currently taking place for cancer of the breast.

Basic methods of study

Epidemiological studies almost always result from some unusual or inexplicable observation. With a disease, ascertainment and descriptions of associations usually start with the collection of a series of cases, the data required being collected from already existing medical records and, if possible, by questioning the patient and his family. This method, the *retrospective* study, is suitable for the investigation of relatively uncommon disease and has the advantage that the required information may be readily available. Care must be taken to ensure that the records available come from a defined population and include all the patients suffering from the condition under study. Further disadvantages are that relevant facts on history or investigations may not be recorded in the case notes and the patients may not be available for questioning or their memory of past events may be faulty.

Many of these problems can be overcome by a *prospective* study in which a population is defined and then followed up so that medical and other associated events are recorded as they happen. The disadvantage of this method is that if a disease occurs infrequently, it will take a considerable number of years to identify sufficient cases to determine significant associations. In addition, some people may be 'lost' through migration or death from a condition other than that being studied. Thus a prospective study is suitable only for common diseases and even then large numbers are needed to compensate for losses. Doll and Hill's study of mortality in registered medical practitioners in relation to their smoking habits is a classic example of a simple and inexpensive prospective study. Doctors' records were 'flagged' and their deaths notified to the epidemiologists as they occurred. Prospective studies may be observational or experimental.

In *observation* or *descriptive* studies, as the name implies, nature is allowed to take its course and changes or differences are merely recorded as and if they occur. Most often such studies are primarily concerned with the amount of a disease or the characteristics of the people with the disease (identification of high-risk groups). Attempts to explain why these people have the disease are sometimes distinguished as *analytic* studies. Occasionally the two stages are tackled together, but in general the hypothesis testing by analytic studies frequently arises out of the suspicions raised in the course of descriptive studies.

With an *experimental* study the investigators actually intervene and change one of the variables under study. A classic example of this approach was the large scale field trials of poliomyelitis vaccine in which two large groups of children comparable in all important respects such as age, health and exposure received vaccine and placebo.

Sampling populations

Very often, it is difficult, impractical or too expensive in time and money to study a complete population (for example, a whole town) and so only a proportion, or *sample*, of the total is studied. There are various methods of obtaining a sample depending on the purpose of the study but the general requirements of a sample are:

(1) that its members should be drawn from the total population in an unbiased way, i.e. each member of the population should have as much chance of becoming a member of the sample as any other member of the population

(2) that the sample should closely resemble the population from which it is drawn in respect of all the characteristics that are considered relevant to the proposed study.

Samples can be drawn to ensure that special or small groups are adequately represented. The commonest of these is the *stratified sample* in which different proportions of some groups (e.g. age groups) are selected. However, even if both these rules are met, it still cannot honestly be claimed that the results of the study apply to the population; they may be distorted in some way that cannot be estimated or even anticipated and thus there is always an element of supposition in the results of any such study.

In some prospective studies there may be a suitable inbuilt comparative group and therefore the need to sample the general population is obviated. Care must be taken, however, to ensure that the composition of the original group did not introduce possible bias. With a retrospective study it is important that any control group meets the above criteria. Particular caution is required in the sometimes tempting situation of comparing the characteristics of patients suffering from one disease with those suffering from other diagnoses thought to be of different aetiology. If sampling is to be carried out, then it is important that it is performed correctly.

Measures of data quality

Observations or measurements, whether made by man or machine, involve some degree of error. Errors affect two important aspects of data quality – validity and reliability.

Validity, or accuracy, is a measure of how closely an observation corresponds to the actual state of affairs. For example, consider a patient with a rapid irregular heartbeat due to atrial fibrillation. Measurement of the heart rate by the radial pulse is considered inaccurate or lacking in validity because some heart beats produce a pulse too weak to be felt at the wrist. Compared to the true heart rate the radial pulse rate is *biased* toward lower values, resulting in what is commonly known as 'pulse deficit'.

Reliability or reproducibility is a measure of how closely a series of observations of exactly the same parameter match one another. If the cholesterol concentration of two portions of the same serum specimen is measured in an autoanalyser, the two results should ideally be exactly the same. If they are not, then the analyser is said to lack reliability.

Rates and ratios

Almost all epidemiological research is concerned with describing the *frequency of events*, whether disease or risk factors, within a population. Since the size of population differs, comparison is easier if these frequencies are expressed in terms of rates.

At its simplest a rate is:

The number of *observed events* divided by the number of *individuals in the population at risk* of experiencing the event

Such rates are usually expressed in terms of each 100 or 1000 of the population since this gives a more manageable figure. A rate must also refer to the period of time over which the events occurred.

For example:

The population of Scotland at a particular mid-year was 5 150 400. In that year there were 63 454 deaths. From this it is possible to calculate

$$\frac{\text{No. of deaths in one year}}{\text{Mid-year population for that year}} = \frac{63\,454}{5\,150\,400}\,(\times\,1000) = 12.32$$

That is, the death rate in Scotland in that particular year was *12.32 deaths per 1000 of the population*. (For details of other rates used in assessing the health of communities *see* pp. 38–9).

Two of the commonest measures in epidemiology are incidence (or inception) and prevalence rates. These two terms have quite different meanings, but are often confused.

An incidence rate refers to the number of new cases of a disease occurring in a population – or the rate of addition. Because this is a rate, the period of time in which this addition takes place and the population at risk must be stated.

Prevalence refers to the number of cases (new or old) in the population at a given time. Because (for almost all conditions) this number is always changing, the period of time for a prevalence must be stated, as *point prevalence* (the number of cases counted *at a given point in time*) or *period prevalence* (the number of cases counted *during a defined period of time*). Prevalence is also usually expressed as a rate per 1000 population at risk. These two types of prevalence have different uses: the former is often difficult to measure but, for example, is used (in conjunction with the incidence rate) to plot an epidemic of an infectious disease. The main value of a period prevalence rate is in chronic disease or for events which occur fairly infrequently. Thus the period prevalence rate for schizophrenia will give a more useful measure of the load placed on the health services by that disease than will its incidence rate.

The death rate given above (p. 16) is a *crude* death rate. While it shows the frequency of deaths in Scotland in a particular year, it is not correct to compare this rate with other death rates (in respect of either time or geography) because the make up (such as age and sex) of other populations will be different. This influences the frequency with which people die and, so that valid comparisons can be made, a device called *standardization* is used.

Briefly, the death rates in various age and sex groups are worked out and are then applied to the same age and sex groups in a selected standard population. This gives a (fictional) rate for that calculation. By repeating the same calculation for deaths from different times or geographical areas, it is possible to obtain other rates that make comparisons valid. Although more usually applied to age and sex, standardization for any attribute or combination of characteristics is possible.

Simple comparisons between rates can be made between similar groups. This is commonly performed by stipulated age and sex categories and these rates are then referred to as *age* (or *sex*) *specific rates*, for example, males aged 45–64. Therefore, breaking down a general rate into a series of specific rates is very useful. Standardized rates are less informative but have the advantage of comparing single figures rather than a series. (For a more detailed explanation of standardization *see* Bradford Hill, 1984, p. 168–182.)

The *standardized mortality ratio (SMR)* is another method of allowing valid comparisons of the number of deaths where there are differences in age, sex, size of population and diseases. The values for each subgroup are calculated as a percentage of the rate occurring in the total population concerned. Thus the standardized mortality ratio for the whole population is 100, subgroups above this value representing a higher risk and those below a lower risk for the disease or geographical area being considered.

HEALTH ECONOMICS

The developing role of epidemiology in studying the effects of treatment was mentioned earlier. While the effectiveness of care is the first concern of doctors and other health professionals, they are becoming increasingly aware that being effective is not enough; we need to try to ensure that care is as effective as possible *given the resources available*.

The shift of emphasis from individuals to populations – essentially a shift from clinical to community medicine – suggests that an appropriate objective ought to be to 'maximize' the health of the population as a whole. Unfortunately, the resources required to bring about improvements in health are finite and will never be sufficient to satisfy all the demands made on them. The need for choice is inescapable and, since choice of how best to use resources is a fundamental concept of, and reason for, the economists' approach, certain economic methods of study are fundamental to planning and evaluating health care. The nature of choice is discussed in Chapter 4 – and, indeed, throughout this Study Guide – but in this chapter the emphasis will be on methods of economic analysis.

Economics considers how society chooses to use its scarce resources to produce various outputs (and about how these outputs are distributed between various users). The resources referred to are items such as labour, equipment and land which are inputs in the production process. Money is not a resource; rather it helps to oil the machinery of an economy by acting as a measure of value and a means of exchange.

Given that resources are scarce, it follows that every time we commit resources to the production of any one output, a sacrifice is involved in that we forgo the output which these resources could have produced in some alternative use (*opportunity cost*). The principle of economic efficiency is that society should make its choices of use of resource in the way that maximizes the value of the total output produced.

Valuation of outputs which are provided in private markets is not a problem as the prices at which they sell often reflect reasonably accurately the values that people attach to them. The more highly they are valued, the more people are willing to pay for them, within the limits of their available funds. Thus prices indicate consumer preferences.

In the case of health, the principle of willingness to pay still applies but, because in the UK people do not have to pay at the point of consumption, we lose price as an indicator of value. Some other way of determining values of health will have to be found if the principle of economic efficiency is to be applied.

Two points require emphasis at this juncture. First, the objective of the health care sector is to provide better health through health services. If a particular programme or policy is not benefiting the people who use it then its output is zero. Services are not provided for their own sake. Yet in many instances we may have to use services (what we call intermediate output) as a proxy measure for final output (health) because the latter cannot be measured at that time. Second, money is used in the analysis as a measure of value, but the cost of producing the health output is seen in terms of the sacrifice incurred (value of output forgone). This is the application of *opportunity cost*.

The idea of weighing the benefits of any programme against the sacrifices which the concept of opportunity cost entails is known as the cost-benefit approach, as shown in Fig. 2.2.

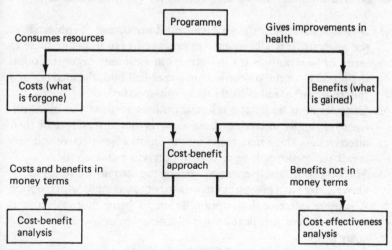

Figure 2.2 The cost-benefit approach (from Drummond, 1980).

As can be seen there are two techniques of appraisal under this approach: cost-effectiveness and cost-benefit analysis.

Cost-effectiveness analysis

Cost-effectiveness analysis is about *how* to do something, given that there are normally alternative ways of realizing any output. It addresses one of two questions: given an objective, which of the alternatives can achieve it at the least cost; or, given a fixed budget, which of the alternatives will yield the greatest benefit? Notice that one alternative cannot be preferred to another solely on the basis of being more effective or solely on the basis of being less costly. The decision must involve both costs and effectiveness.

The term 'cost-effective' is frequently misused; for example, particular policies are declared to be cost-effective. Strictly this has no meaning. Since cost-effectiveness analysis seeks only to find the preferred alternative among those identified, one of them must emerge as being the *most* cost-effective. Cost-effectiveness is thus a relative state and no policy can be cost-effective in any absolute sense. It follows that cost-effectiveness analysis does not directly help in addressing the questions of whether the chosen objective is worth pursuing at all or, if so, to what extent.

Cost-effectiveness analysis ideally requires four factors to be considered (although many such studies fall short of the ideal).

(1) A clear statement of the problem and the nature of the objective of the analysis. It is all too easy in practice to fail to define these in terms of final outputs (i.e. reductions in morbidity or mortality). If the problem or the objective is mis-specified both the analysis and the 'solution' are also likely to be mis-specified.
(2) Consideration of all the relevant options to meet the objective. Clearly, simply analysing those most favoured in terms of their effectiveness alone may mean that the most cost-effective solution is not recommended, since that option was not analysed.
(3) The extent of effectiveness of each of the options (in terms of (1) above). Here it is important to quantify the extent to which option A is more effective than option B. Simply being more effective is not a sufficient justification for choosing option A, unless it also costs less.
(4) Cost data: such costs will include all costs that arise as a result of

implementing the options, no matter on whom the costs fall – patients, relatives of patients, other public sector and private sector agencies. Measurement of these may well prove difficult, but they should at least be described lest their complete omission results in an implicit 'zero value' being attached to them.

An example of a cost-effectiveness analysis was the investigation on breast cancer screening which examined 11 alternatives to an existing screening regimen. At the time of the study, all women who attended the screening clinic were given mammography, thermography (with double reporting of the results), and two physical examinations. The total cost of running the clinic for a year was £63 000 and the total number of women screened was 3857. Thus the cost per woman screened was £16.50 as shown in Table 2.1.

Table 2.1 *Screening costs per woman screened under different screening regimens*

	Double reporting (£)	Single reporting (£)
(1) Mammography, thermography + 2 PEs	16.50	15.80
(2) Thermography + 2 PEs	13.50	13.00
(3) Mammography + 2 PEs	13.50	13.20
(4) Mammography, thermography + 1 PE	14.60	13.90
(5) Thermography + 1 PE	11.70	11.20
(6) Mammography + 1 PE	11.60	11.30

PE: physical examination
(From Mooney, 1982)

The alternatives considered are also shown in Table 2.1 together with the associated cost per woman screened. The cheapest alternative is thermography with single reporting and one physical examination. This Table, however, does not provide enough information to find the most cost-effective alternative for several reasons.

First, Table 2.1 concerns costs only and says nothing about effectiveness. Screening is not carried out for its own sake. Rather it is done in order to detect presymptomatic cancer, where presymptomatic detection will improve the effectiveness or cost of subsequent treatment. The most cost-effective alternative will be that with the lowest cost per cancer detected, not the lowest cost per woman screened.

Second, detecting a case of cancer involves more than just screening costs. For example, various alternatives can have different numbers of positive screening results.

Since all positive results, true or false, are sent for biopsy we would thus need to include the cost of biopsy in the cost of each alternative. We would also want to include non-money costs such as the anxiety associated with a false positive. (Note that costs which do not affect the ranking of alternatives can be ignored.)

This analysis does not directly provide any assistance in deciding whether or not screening for breast cancer represents an efficient use of resources. To do that requires cost-benefit analysis.

Cost-benefit analysis

Cost-benefit analysis concerns the *whether* of policy, and stresses the simple point that it is only worth doing something if the advantage gained justifies the sacrifice involved. It is all too easy to argue that life is priceless and no effort should be spared when lives are at risk. Such thinking, while understandable at the level of an individual patient, leads to inefficiency and less overall health from the available resources than could otherwise be obtained. If we spend large sums of money to save life in one way, we inevitably forgo benefits elsewhere. The issues that cost-benefit analysis force us to consider are not only what to do, but what to leave undone.

Where many find cost-benefit analysis objectionable is at the level of placing monetary values on both the costs and the benefits, and particularly the latter, of health care policies. If we are genuinely to compare disadvantages and advantages on the same measuring rod and since costs are frequently expressed in money terms, then it becomes desirable to measure the benefits—reduced mortality and morbidity for example – in money terms. But how can this be done? Is it necessary? Is it ethical?

The first answer is that it is not necessary; it only becomes necessary if it is believed that an efficient NHS is a good thing, and an efficient NHS means attempting to ensure that the health obtainable is maximized from available resources. If we are content to fall short of doing the most in terms of 'providing health', then efficiency or cost-benefit analysis are not of interest.

Rather than asking if cost-benefit analysis is ethical, it seems more appropriate to ask if it is ethical to fail to do as much as we can from the resources available to the NHS to promote health. That, in essence, is what cost-benefit analysis seeks to do. Yet even if it is accepted that cost-benefit analysis is desirable and ethical, can a monetary value be placed on such health outputs as reduced pain and suffering, or even human life? Certainly attempts have been made to do so, some quite sophisticated, some simple minded. However, the question is irrelevant. There is no question of whether or not we can place a value on such intangibles; the fact is that we do every time a decision is taken which involves allocating or not allocating scarce resources in health care.

Say, for example, we are considering an immunization programme against some particular disease. The costs of the programme are simply the value of all the resources used, including the value of the time of the consumers who come forward for the immunization. Let us say the total cost comes to £100 000. The benefits of the programme are those associated with fewer cases of the disease. Let us assume that 50 cases are prevented. Some of the associated benefits, such as the resources which will not be used to treat these 50 cases or the reduction in sickness absence from work due to less illness, can be fairly easily expressed in monetary terms. Say this totals £60 000. This leaves a net cost of £40 000 and the question can then be put: 'are the benefits of reduced pain, suffering, etc., from 50 avoided cases of this disease worth at least £40 000 (given the notion of opportunity cost)?' If the answer is 'yes', then the programme passes the cost-benefit test.

Many resource expenditures are approved or rejected without the use of economic appraisal. In all such cases, values are implied in the decisions taken. Valuation is thus unavoidable. Cost-benefit analysis seeks to make these values explicit to assist the pursuit of efficiency. (For a detailed introduction to cost-benefit analysis and some practical applications *see* Drummond, 1980.)

Marginal analysis

Cost-benefit analysis is concerned not only with the issue of whether or not to pursue any policy, but also with the question of *how much*? When considering expanding or contracting any programme the relevant questions are 'what are the extra costs (savings)?' and 'what are the extra benefits (losses)?' Total costs and benefits, and average costs and benefits are irrelevant to the expansion or contraction question. Say, for example, that care for the mentally handicapped is provided in hospitals and also in the community, and at present £9 million is spent on the hospital section and £1 million in the community. To examine whether or not we are maximizing the total benefit from this overall £10 million expenditure on care of the mentally handicapped we would want to examine what would happen if we did more of one type of care and less of the other. If £100 000 were taken away from the hospital sector, there would be a loss of benefit (sacrifice). If that £100 000 were then spent in the community sector, there would be an increase in benefit (gain). While the value judgment cannot be avoided, the question is now whether or not the sacrifice is judged to be greater or less than the gain. If greater, then no switch should be made; if less, then we should make the switch, since overall total benefit will be increased. We should continue transferring blocks of expenditure in one direction or the other until a position is reached where the benefit lost by the decreased expenditure in the one programme exactly equals the benefit gained by the increased expenditure in the other programme. Notice that the average cost (or benefit) of care in either regimen is irrelevant to this decision.

An example that highlights the usefulness of marginal costs over the more commonly used average costs is the American Cancer Society's recommendations for a screening programme for presymptomatic cancer of the colon. A protocol of six sequential examinations for faecal occult blood was suggested.

This number of tests overcomes the high false negative rate of 8.33% and ensures that 99.99% of all cancers of the colon are detected during the full screening programme. In a population of 100 million some 720 000 cases can be expected. The average cost for each cancer found in this programme – which includes, of course, the cost of diagnosis in addition to screening – was given as $2451.

However, if one uses marginal cost analysis or the cost for each additional case of cancer detected at every stage of screening, costs look very different. As can be seen from Table 2.2 the first screening round, which yields 659 469 cases (91.67% of 720 000), costs $1175 per case detected. Screening all negatives once more will yield 54 956; with each successive screening the yield of new positive cases decreases so that by the sixth round of tests only three additional cases are detected at a cost of $47 107 214 each.

Table 2.2 *Incremental cases detected and incremental and marginal costs ($) of sequential faecal occult blood tests*

Number of sets of tests	Additional cases detected at each screening	Marginal cost* ($)
1	659 469	1175
2	54 956	5492
3	4580	49 150
4	382	469 534
5	32	4 724 695
6	3	47 107 214

*The marginal cost is the incremental cost divided by the incremental cases detected (that is, it is the additional cost of the nth test divided by the additional cases detected by the nth test).

The American Cancer Society can now ask itself the question: 'is it worth paying over $47M to detect one case of colonic cancer, given the notion of opportunity cost?' If the answer is 'no', then the next question is: 'is it worth paying $4.7M (the marginal cost in the fifth test)?' Once a judgement is reached that it is worth paying the marginal cost, then that determines the number of sets of tests to conduct.

In screening programmes such as this example it is relatively easy to identify the costs of using additional tests and the yield from screening additional groups of people with different levels of risk.

Most other policy decisions are much more complex. Nevertheless, in the context of the NHS, similar analyses of policy options can be conducted. In this way decision-making becomes more explicit and, eventually, more rational. The rationality will follow when sufficient studies are mounted that the marginal costs of similar outputs can be equated across different policy areas.

In any system of planning resources, judgement is needed. Marginal analysis persuades the decision-maker to exercise his judgement about the right 'area', i.e. at the margin, and forces the decision-maker to be explicit about the weights he attaches to one type of output as opposed to another. While not perfect, it can be of assistance in deploying scarce health care resources by focusing on the precise groups of patients who would be affected by an increase or decrease in a particular service. It is then easier for most people to put relative values on which patients would benefit most or suffer least – easier in one sense because it is clearer, but more difficult in that the losers are identified. This highlights what is perhaps the most important concept that the economic approach offers, namely opportunity cost.

However, we cannot assume efficiency in health care. Encouragement, motivation and the provision of the right 'carrots and sticks' are needed to promote efficiency. Indeed, it is only recently that the NHS has begun to think seriously about the concept of clinical budgeting and other mechanisms to make clinicians more aware of the resources they use and their cost and thereby encourages them to be more efficient. At present there is little incentive to clinicians to look beyond effectiveness. Yet that is not enough if the goal of maximizing the health of the population from the resources available is to be achieved.

The economic approach is, thus, not primarily about money. When an economic evaluation concludes that benefit X is not worth cost Y, it means simply that there is some alternative use of Y which could give benefits judged to be of greater value than X. If we agree that greater value is better, then clearly the pursuit of X is not wise. The economic approach is primarily concerned with weighing gains and sacrifices. This way of thinking can be of much assistance to planning the efficient use of health care resources even when there are problems involved in applying the techniques.

INFORMATION SERVICES

As discussed later in this chapter it can be misleading to use information to answer one question when it was originally collected for a different purpose. However, much of the information that is used to answer questions of mortality, population and use of services is applied in the same way each time. It has, therefore, been possible and useful to build up a routine system of data collection which is justified by the frequency of its use.

A health information service provides the data required for all relevant health service purposes including patient care, management, planning, evaluation and research which may be clinical, operational or epidemiological. To function properly, information services must be concerned with the manner in which data are originally recorded in clinical records or in administrative offices; its collection in a

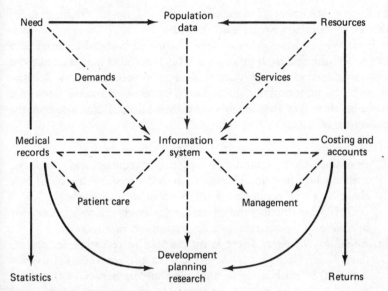

Figure 2.3 Health information system.

structured and ordered form; and making it available in a useful and understandable form.

The *sources of information* for epidemiological studies are listed on pp. 34–6, but for evaluation of clinical care and of health services, and for planning purposes, a more extensive database is required. A diagrammatic representation of such a system is shown in Fig. 2.3. The input of information on *patients* and the demands which they currently make on the services is mainly derived by extraction of summary data from case records. For example, in Scotland, a Scottish Morbidity Return (SMR form) is completed for all hospital discharges. The content of clinical information for each type of hospital varies from SMR1 (for general hospital discharges), where only diagnoses and operations are recorded, to SMR2 (maternity hospital discharges) which includes details of antenatal complications, labour, puerperium and of the baby. In England and Wales, the national Hospital In-Patient Enquiry system (HIPE) comprises data on a 10% random sample of discharges and deaths, while Hospital Activity Analysis (HAA) includes all such discharges, but is not available on a national basis. Annual publications from OPCS (Hospital In-Patient Enquiry – Main Tables) and, in Scotland, SHIPS (Scottish Hospital

In-Patient Statistics) give details of the diagnostic distribution of discharges for each Area Health Board.

However, as discussed elsewhere, the use of hospital facilities may not reflect the real need in an area. This latter may be obtained from well-organized general practice records or by special surveys. Because most of the information collected on patients is abstracted from case records, there are two areas where medical staff can assist in the collection of data:

(1) *Recording of information.* Case notes must be legible and it is desirable that these should be filed in a set sequence and contain all relevant information. The use of standardized or structured case sheets is to be commended. Problem orientated medical records (POMR) are one method of making relevant information readily available to those extracting data from the case records.

(2) *Reliability of data.* There is no purpose in recording inaccurate data. Every attempt must be made to ensure accuracy. Errors may occur (a) by mishearing or misunderstanding between patient and recorder (ensure patient understands any medical terms being used); (b) when writing information into a case record (more likely to occur if recording is done some time after history-taking); (c) in copying information from one form or record sheet to another (copying should be reduced to a minimum).

Population data are obtained from the Decennial Census carried out by the Office of Population Censuses and Surveys in England and Wales and the Registrar General in Scotland. The most recent Census, held in 1981, included details such as age, sex, marital status and occupations of the population of each area. By taking account of births, deaths and migration into and out of an area, population estimates for intercensal years and population projections for the future are also provided. This latter is of considerable value in planning, for example, services for the elderly.

In an information system it is also important to include details of the health service *resources* which are available in an area, and to relate these to the population served and the patients using the services. These resources are of three main types:

(1) *Physical resources.* For example number of beds available to each speciality and their distribution between various hospitals; location of x-ray machines and their likely replacement date.

(2) *Manpower*. The number of all types and grades of staff. Again national returns are completed for this and published annually.
(3) *Finance*. Information is obtained from various returns. In the past the data published related mainly to broad categories such as 'cost per hospital bed per week', but these are becoming increasingly specific to enable, for example, a cost to be ascribed to a particular service (e.g. child health), to a speciality (e.g. ophthalmology) and to the drugs used in a particular ward.

Annual publications (Health and Personal Social Services Statistics for England, HMSO and Scottish Health Statistics, HMSO) give summary information on these various resources. In fact, these publications are recommended as a good starting point for any enquiry for data relating to the health services.

Thus an *information system* comprises:

(1) annual reports and various statistical returns
(2) computer file (usually of patient based information)
(3) knowledge of, and access to, specialized reports or returns in the various departments of the NHS.

Although most information is held at, and reports published from, national level, in recent years there has been a development by health authorities of information systems at local level. Thus, in the first instance, anyone (staff or student) requiring information is encouraged to find out what is available locally, as this may well be more detailed and more up-to-date than can be obtained nationally. In addition, and most importantly, advice will be available on the most appropriate data to use for specific purposes and on its interpretation.

The uses of the *output* of an information system are also indicated in Fig. 2.3. In addition to the various statistical returns produced, the system can be used to assist in patient care, management and planning, and research.

Patient care

The clinician can use the information service to improve individual patient care. Feedback of information can be either routine (as in returns made to each consultant so that he can compare his workload with that of all other colleagues in the area and nationally in terms of diagnoses, age, length of stay, i.e. peer review) or *ad hoc* (where the information given is designed to answer a specific query by the clinician).

Management and planning

The uses for this purpose are discussed elsewhere in this chapter in Evaluation below and Economics (p. 18). Simple information on trends in particular diagnostic patterns can often be of considerable value in estimating future requirements. This can assist in short-term management as well as long-term planning. In using data for these, it is important not only to take account of the statistics themselves, but also the manner in which they have been collected and any other changes which are not being measured but which may have an important effect on any trends observed, e.g. new therapeutic developments.

Research

To some extent this overlaps with the use of data in planning, but it should be remembered that in addition to epidemiological research, the information system can assist in clinical research. Thus patients with a specified diagnosis or from a particular town can be identified and a computer list provided.

AN EVALUATIVE FRAMEWORK

It may be helpful to emphasize that the terms 'valuation' and 'evaluation' have different meanings. The Oxford English Dictionary distinguishes them by the extent to which they reflect subjective and objective assessments as follows:

Valuation: the appreciation or estimation of something in respect of excellence or merit.
Evaluation: the ascertainment of the amount of; expression in terms of the known.

Thus, valuation is a single subjective act, but evaluation is a process of bringing together relevant factual information in a way which allows measurement. Values and data are both part of evaluation.

Epidemiology and economics are two evaluative approaches which have slightly different objectives – epidemiology to understand causes of disease and thereby improve methods of treatment; economics to understand delivery of treatment and thereby improve its output – but both have the ultimate aim of achieving the greatest possible improvement in the health state of a group or a community with the skills and resources available.

It is possible to fit these and other evaluative approaches into a common framework which can be used for virtually any problem analysis in health and medical care. It is this framework which is of most use to doctors and others in deciding which patients to treat and how best to do it.

A few people may still ask why a formalized approach to such choices is necessary. Perhaps the most important reason is that not everyone has the same underlying aims or values which shape their choices, yet these values influence the kinds of questions that we ask ourselves in deciding what is 'good' care or health for any patient or community. Much of the argument and uncertainty within medicine arises because people who work together do not spell out (indeed, may not be aware of) their different aims and values. This affects several aspects of medicine – continuity of care between doctors and other team members; basic and continuing education of students and staff; and choices of priorities. While records, journals and committees all help in the exchange of information, many decisions are taken outside this network. The first step in any evaluative exercise is, therefore, a statement of objectives so that the subsequent questions are directed to these objectives and do not, as so often happens, lead to irrelevant answers.

The framework for evaluating an aspect of clinical care rests on three sets of information.

(1) A statement of objectives – *what are we trying to achieve*? Measures of improving the health of a patient may be made in terms of saving life, decreasing disease and disability, and restoring independence (mental, physical and social). The same types of measures may be sought for a population, e.g. fatality rates for a particular disease, percentage of the population who are handicapped, duration of time off work, incidence of preventable infectious disease. The most relevant of these measures of *outcome* of care should be chosen to compare the impact of a particular treatment

or service. For example, there is no point in trying to evaluate a
service used mainly by elderly people by its impact on time off
work. However, before judging the effect, it is necessary to know
the starting point from which to measure.

(2) Definition and ascertainment of the problem and how it is being
handled – *what is happening now*? Description and measurement
of what is happening may be patients' signs and symptoms; the
population's disease characteristics (descriptive epidemiology); the
availability and use of services; or indicators of mortality and
morbidity. The corresponding techniques of collecting and presenting this information include the format of medical records;
retrospective and prospective epidemiological studies; health
service statistics of facilities, expenditure and use of services;
population statistics of births, sickness and deaths.

(3) List of feasible options or alternative approaches, with benefits
and costs identified and measured where possible – *what is the
best way to reach our objectives*? The choice of what is 'best' is the
essence of economic evaluation. It incorporates the criteria of
effectiveness, efficiency and acceptability.

  (a) *Effectiveness* should be measured in terms of the relevant
  outcomes, referred to in (1) above. Techniques of comparing
  the effectiveness of different options include 'before and after'
  studies, and randomized controlled clinical trials.

  (b) *Efficiency* is the comparison of the effort or resources used in
  different ways to achieve the same effect (usually called cost-
  effectiveness analysis). It is important because if the most
  efficient treatment is chosen, then more people can benefit
  with the same amount of effort. Operational research is a
  technique often used to test for more efficient ways of
  providing health services.

  (c) *Acceptability* is less objective than effectiveness and efficiency,
  but is just as important. It concerns the values of patients, staff
  and society about what is 'good' care. The techniques of
  finding out about acceptability are, mainly, to ask those
  concerned or to analyse previous experience of particular
  treatments or services.

Ideally, all the benefits or outcomes (including the nature of factors
which influence acceptability) are then set against all the costs of a
treatment or service (including the costs to the patients and families) to

allow a cost-benefit analysis. Often, all the benefits and costs cannot be measured, but they can be described. If it can be assumed that some are approximately the same in the various options, then they cancel each other out. The analysis then is only of the factors which are known to differ, giving a relative rather than an absolute result. If the benefits are thought to be the same in all options then the analysis becomes one of costs only.

The *evaluation of priorities* is to see whether resources are distributed across the many and varied groups likely to benefit in a way which produces the maximum improvement in the health state of the community being served. (The economists' term is distributional or allocative efficiency – not to be confused with clinical efficiency.) It rests on the question: 'how much of each service can we afford to provide?', and the approach is to compare the marginal groups of patients in each service or programme who would actually be affected by an increase or decrease in that service (*see* p. 23). In principle the *net* marginal benefits (strictly, the ratios of marginal benefit to marginal cost) from each programme should all be equal. In practice, measures of benefit are often missing, but at least by this approach the right patients are being compared when judgements are made about the balance between services.

One particular application of the evaluative framework is nowadays receiving increasing attention, namely, the examination of their own work by groups of doctors. It is known as *peer review* or *medical audit*. The Committee of Inquiry into Competence to Practise (1976) characterized medical audit as 'the sharing by a group of peers of information gained from personal experience and/or medical records in order to assess the care provided to their patients, to improve their learning and to contribute to medical knowledge'. The Committee understood the term 'peer group' to mean a group of doctors who practise in the same speciality and under broadly similar conditions, and they believed that it is a necessary part of a doctor's professional responsibility to assess his work regularly with his colleagues.

One of the first and best known examples is the confidential enquiry into maternal deaths, which began in England and Wales in 1952 and which has since reported regularly. However, there are many approaches to peer review; it may involve simple reporting of the variation in, say, use of laboratory investigations or it may compare doctors' clinical practice against a predetermined minimum standard of activity or outcome. Whatever the method used, the aim is clearly stated as educational and non-punitive and all the postgraduate colleges promote its development as an integral part of doctors' work.

There are many articles on peer review in medical journals, often using the term 'quality of care' (*see* References, p. 42).

Finally, when trying to judge whether a published study is valid, the following set of questions brings together the main issues of epidemiology and evaluation and is in itself a useful evaluative framework.

(1) What was the main question being asked?
(2) What was the hypothesis?
(3) What method was used to collect the data?
(4) What population was sampled?
(5) What were the variables important to the study?
(6) How were these tested (briefly)?
(7) What results were found?
(8) What was the author's conclusion?
(9) Did it answer the question?

MAIN SOURCES OF HEALTH CARE INFORMATION

Certificates

(1) Birth certificates
(2) Death certificates
Each birth and death is registered locally and the information is sent to the Office of Population Censuses and Surveys for England and Wales or the Registrar General for Scotland. Annual reports are produced giving detailed analyses and tabulations.
(3) Department of Health and Social Security Certificates of incapacity for work and of industrial injury. (Since these certificates may be seen both by patient and employer the diagnostic information contained is of variable validity.)

Notification

(1) Certain specified infectious diseases (to the appropriate Medical Officer of the local health authority, published in weekly reports, *see* p. 36)

(2) Certain other diseases in specific localities (to the appropriate Medical Officer of the local health authority)

(3) Food poisoning (to the appropriate Medical Officer of the local health authority)

(4) Certain specified industrial diseases and accidents (to Health and Safety Executive).

Medical records

(1) Hospital
  (a) *Case record folders*: general, maternity, psychiatric.
  (b) *Abstracts*: Morbidity returns: HIPE; HAA; SMR (*see* p. 27). Cancer registration – each new case of malignant disease is registered so that incidence and survival can be calculated.
  (c) *Statistical returns of admissions, discharges,* etc. (reports derived from (b) above)
(2) General practice
(3) Community health departments of health authorities
  maternal and child health
  school health service
  handicapped persons
(4) Certain industries and occupations
  armed services
  British Rail
  Post Office
  National Coal Board
  large companies such as ICI and Unilever
(5) Health and Safety Executive: Employment Medical Advisory Service Records of all employees in hazardous occupations, e.g. chrome plating, lead processing.

Special surveys

(1) Research units of central government departments
(2) Medical Research Council epidemiological units (e.g. case finding in total population in the Rhondda Valley, South Wales)
(3) University epidemiological units
(4) Local health authority epidemiological units
(5) Social surveys division of the Office of Population Censuses and Surveys (especially general household survey)

(6) Royal College of General Practitioners epidemiological research units
(7) Independent units, e.g. Institute of Community Studies
(8) The actuarial departments of life insurance companies.

The decennial and sample censuses

These provide the population denominators for national and local studies together with data on occupation, marital state, family size and housing.

Environmental data

This is obtained from:

(1) the Meteorological Office
(2) environmental health departments of local government authorities (records of atmospheric pollution levels, etc.)
(3) the geological department of Ordnance Survey (for the presence of trace elements or certain strata that contribute to background radiation, etc.)

World Health Organization epidemiological data

This is useful for comparative purposes.

For further information on all sources *see* Alderson M. (1983) *An Introduction to Epidemiology*, Chapter 3. London: Macmillan Press.

NOTIFIABLE DISEASES

Regulations require that the following infectious diseases be notified to the appropriate medical officer of the local health authority on a prescribed form. For the more serious diseases, notification by telephone prior to the despatch of written notification is requested, but not obligatory. This is usually done by the general practitioner or hospital doctor who makes the diagnosis, and who receives a fee for each notification:

† Acute meningitis
Anthrax
Cholera
* Continued fever
Diphtheria
Dysentery
† Encephalitis
* Erysipelas
Food poisoning
† Infective jaundice
Lassa fever
Leprosy
Leptospiral jaundice
Malaria
Marburg disease
Measles
* Meningococcal infection
Ophthalmia neonatorum

Paratyphoid (A and B)
Plague
Poliomyelitis
* Puerperal fever
Rabies
Relapsing fever
** Rubella
Scarlet fever
Smallpox
† Tetanus
Tuberculosis
Typhoid fever
Typhus fever
Viral haemorrhagic fever
* Viral hepatitis
Whooping cough
Yellow fever

† England and Wales only
* Scotland only
** Edinburgh and Glasgow only

The Health and Safety at Work legislation and subsequent regulations require every medical practitioner to notify the Health and Safety Executive of the following diseases if believed to have been contracted in the course of work:

Aniline poisoning
Anthrax
Arsenical poisoning
Beryllium poisoning
Cadmium poisoning
Carbon bisulphide poisoning
Chrome ulceration
Chronic benzene poisoning

Compressed air sickness
Epitheliomatous ulceration
Lead poisoning
Manganese poisoning
Mercurial poisoning
Phosphorus poisoning
Toxic anaemia
Toxic jaundice

Regulations made under the Misuse of Drugs Act, 1971, require that any doctor who attends a person whom he considers, or has reasonable grounds to suspect, is addicted to any drug shall, within 7 days of the attendance, furnish in writing to the chief medical officer at the Home Office the name, address, sex, date of birth, NHS number of the patient and the name of the drug or drugs concerned.

ASSESSING THE HEALTH OF A COMMUNITY

Various rates are used in assessing the health of communities. In calculating rates the numerator (number of events) and the denominator (population at risk) must refer to the same area (e.g. country or town), and comparable year.

Birth rate

$$\frac{\text{Number of live births}}{\text{Total mid-year population}} \times 1000$$

Total fertility rate

$$\frac{\text{Number of live births}}{\text{Number of women aged 15–44 years}} \times 1000$$

Crude death rate

$$\frac{\text{Number of deaths}}{\text{Total mid-year population}} \times 1000$$

Age-specific death rate

$$\frac{\text{Number of deaths of persons of specified age}}{\text{Number of persons in the population in the same age group}} \times 1000$$

Cause-specific death rate

$$\frac{\text{Number of deaths attributed to a specified cause of death}}{\text{Total mid-year population}} \times 1000$$

Age- and cause-specific death rates

$$\frac{\text{Number of deaths of persons of specified age attributed to a specified cause}}{\text{Number of persons in the population in the same age group}} \times 1000$$

Infant mortality rate

$$\frac{\text{Number of deaths of infants in the first year of life}}{\text{Number of live births}} \times 1000$$

Neonatal mortality rate

$$\frac{\text{Number of deaths of infants in the first 4 weeks of life}}{\text{Number of live births}} \times 1000$$

Perinatal mortality rate

$$\frac{\text{Number of still births} + \text{deaths in first week of life}}{\text{Total births (live and still)}} \times 1000$$

Still-birth rate

$$\frac{\text{Number of still births}}{\text{Total number of births (live and still)}} \times 1000$$

INTERNATIONAL VARIATIONS IN DISEASE

Although there is little information about morbidity in many parts of the world and even mortality data may be unreliable, the World Health Organization has, through its International Classification of Disease (ICD), contributed much to standardize methods of recording. Thus it has become possible to compare death rates for different countries and these are published regularly in the World Health Statistics Annual. Caution must always be exercised, however, in the interpretation of such statistics since, for example, there are international differences in the form of death certification, in the proportion of deaths in a given country certified by qualified medical practitioners, in the availability of diagnostic facilities and in the use of different terminology for identical symptoms and signs.

Certain differences are at once obvious. For example, in countries with a low standard of living and high mortality such as India, infectious diseases are the major cause of mortality and cancer and ischaemic heart disease are not among the 'major killers'. In countries with a high standard of living and low mortality as in the UK and USA, ischaemic heart disease and cancer are the main causes of death.

Some factors which may account for international variation in disease incidence are listed below:

Climate

The mosquito, which causes malaria, requires particular breeding conditions (including a minimum temperature) and the disease is, therefore, limited to those areas where such conditions prevail.

Socio-economic state

In the UK the mortality from infectious disease fell markedly in the first quarter of the twentieth century as a consequence of the improved living standards, (e.g. housing, sanitation, nutrition) associated with a general improved socio-economic status. It is probable that as other countries become industrialized, they will go through the same pattern of changing mortality and morbidity, but the change will be more rapid and will be modified by knowledge and attitudes picked up from industrial countries as part of general international exchange.

Nature and nurture

It has frequently been suggested that certain races appear to have a genetic predisposition for a particular condition and yet there is little concrete evidence to support this. More frequently than not, the racial differences are associated with social and environmental factors rather than genetic differences. For example, the mortality in Scotland from ischaemic heart disease and cancer is notably higher than in Sweden, although the two countries lie at similar latitudes. The populations, which are of similar size differ considerably in their smoking, drinking, eating and exercise habits and Scotland is more industrialized than Sweden. Such differences are more likely to be important in the aetiology of these diseases than genetic factors.

REFERENCES AND FURTHER READING

There is no one textbook which fully covers all aspects. The essential chapters in recommended textbooks are indicated in the lists below. Also included is a range of further sources depending on the particular issue that individual students may wish to pursue. If seeking information on a particular subject, the reference list at the end of *Uses of Epidemiology*, Morris, 1975, p. 284 *et seq.* is one of the most useful starting points that can be found.

Epidemiology
Introduction
Any of these four will provide a suitable introduction and the differences between them is merely in detail.

Alderson M. (1983) *An Introduction to Epidemiology*. London: Macmillan

Farmer R. D. T., Miller D. L. (1983) *Lecture Notes on Epidemiology and Community Medicine*, pp. 1–57. Oxford: Blackwell

Roberts C. J. (1977) *Epidemiology for Clinicians*, pp. 3–154. London: Pitman Medical

Rose G., Barker D. J. P. (1979) *Epidemiology for the Uninitiated*. London: British Medical Association

Sampling and standardization
Bradford Hill A. (1984) *A Short Textbook of Medical Statistics*. London: Hodder and Stoughton

Specific conditions
Doll R. (1967) *Prevention of Cancer; Pointers from Epidemiology*, pp. 15–91. London: Nuffield Provincial Hospitals Trust

Doll R., Hill A. B. (1964) Mortality in relation to smoking: ten years' experience of British doctors. *British Medical Journal*, i, 1399–1410; 1460–7

Medical Commission on Accident Prevention (1972) *Medical Aspects of Home Hazards*. London: Medical Commission on Accident Prevention, (Report)

Morris J. N. (1975) *Uses of Epidemiology*. pp. 142–249. Edinburgh: Churchill Livingstone

Office of Health Economics (1977) *Preventing Bronchitis*. London: HMSO (Paper no. 59)

Health economics
Drummond M. F. (1980) *Principles of Economic Appraisal in Health Care*. Oxford: Oxford Medical

Mooney G. H., Russell E. M., Weir R. D. (1986) *Choices for Health Care*. London: Macmillan

Williams A., Anderson R. (1975) *Efficiency in the Social Services.*
Oxford: Basil Blackwell & Martin Robertson

Health information services

Alderson M. (1983) *An Introduction to Epidemiology*, pp. 45–88.
London: Macmillan

Farmer R. D. T., Miller D. L. (1983) *Lecture Notes on Epidemiology
and Community Medicine*, pp. 58–87. Oxford: Blackwell

World Health Organization. (1977) *Health Services: Concepts and
Information for National Planning and Management.* Geneva:
WHO (Public Health Paper No. 67.)

Health services research and evaluation

Barker D. J. P., Rose G. (1984) *Epidemiology in Medical Practice*, pp.
142–150. Edinburgh: Churchill Livingstone

Holland W. W., Gilderdale S. (1977) *Epidemiology and Health*,
pp.11–28. London: Kimpton

Morris J. N. (1975) *Uses of Epidemiology*, pp. 71–97. Edinburgh:
Churchill Livingstone

Quality of care

Brooke R. H., Appel F. A. (1973) Quality of care assessment: choosing
a method for peer review. *New England Journal of Medicine* **288**:
1323–29

Committee of Inquiry into Competence to Practise. (1976) *Report.*
(Alment E. A. J. Chairman). London

Fowkes F. G. R., Evans R. C., Williams L. A., Gehlbach S. H., Cooke
B. R. B., Roberts C. J. (1984) Implementation of guidelines for the
use of skull radiographs in patients with head injury. *Lancet* **ii**:
795–7

Scottish Council for Postgraduate Medical Education. (1981) *Maintaining Standards in General Practice.* Edinburgh: Scottish Council
for Postgraduate Medical Education

Shaw C. D. (1980) Aspects of audit. *British Medical Journal* **i**:
1256–8; 1314–6; 1361–3; 1443–6; 1509–11

Specific articles

Buxton M. J., West R. R. (1975) Cost benefit analysis of longterm
haemodialysis for chronic renal failure. *British Medical Journal* **ii**:
376–9

Culyer A. J., Maynard A. K. (1981) Cost effectiveness of duodenal
ulcer treatment. *Social Science and Medicine*, **15C**: 3–11

Mooney G. H. (1982) Breast cancer screening: a study in cost-
effectiveness analysis. *Social Science and Medicine* **16**: 1277–83

Piachaud D., Weddell J. (1972) The economics of treating varicose veins. *International Journal of Epidemiology*, 1: 3

Simpson P. R., Chamberlain J., Gravelle H. (1978) Choice of screening tests. *Journal of Epidemiology and Community Health*, 32: 166–70

Williams A. (1979) One economist's view of social medicine. *Journal of Epidemiology and Community Health*, 33: 3–7

Wright K. C. (1979) Measurement of costs and benefits in health and health services. *Journal of Epidemiology and Community Health*, 33: 19–31

Chapter

3

Prevention

OUTLINE • PRIMARY PREVENTION • SECONDARY PREVENTION •
TERTIARY PREVENTION AND REHABILITATION • HEALTH EDUCATION
• ENVIRONMENTAL HEALTH CONTROL • HEALTH AT WORK •
INTERNATIONAL HEALTH ORGANIZATIONS

The role of international health organizations is largely preventive and
hence it has been included in this chapter. International health care
systems themselves are described in Chapter 4. Further discussions of
the general principles and examples are given in the Further reading
list on p. 80. The preventive philosophy means actively looking for
trouble before patients present with a problem. Prevention is said to be
better than cure. Despite this our commitment to prevention is small
since less than 5% of the NHS budget is spent on prevention. Control
of infectious diseases has been achieved by applying effective
preventive programmes within both health and other statutory
services such as housing and sanitation, and much of prevention is still
directed toward that end. In this last quarter of the twentieth century
when degenerative diseases are of increasing importance and our
expectation of life is barely increasing, it is vital that we should
seriously consider the current contribution made by the preventive
approach, examine its relevance and see how it can be made more
effective. If prevention is not only better but also cheaper than cure, it
may, in the end, release resources which can then be used for those
individuals whose diseases are less amenable to prevention. However,
prevention will always have to compete for resources with acute care,
which usually shows a quicker return from action. Therefore
prevention will only become widespread when information to evaluate
preventive measures is routinely available and they are thereby shown
to be effective.

Because prevention applies usually to people who feel well,
individual freedom of choice is a more overt issue than in ill patients
and, even if objective evidence of benefit exists, it may be outweighed

by other values within society. An example would be the past reluctance of government to enforce the use of seat belts, not on economic grounds but because it would be seen as an unacceptable level of interference with personal choice of behaviour. Preventive approaches can be taken by everyone involved in health care and there is no single preventive service. However, health visitors and health education officers are specifically trained to practise and promote prevention. This chapter introduces the philosophy and techniques of prevention and draws together the various facets of prevention which you will meet during the course of your medical studies.

OBJECTIVES

Students should know:

(1) that prevention depends to a large extent on knowing the natural history of disease
(2) the principles of primary and secondary prevention
(3) the arrangements for provision of preventive services, including health education, and the role of the primary care team in preventing disease, both in children and in adults; the current position of immunization against communicable diseases and the method of evaluating the costs and benefits of an immunization programme
(4) examples of medical problems for which behaviour change is the main solution and of others in which legislation has played an important preventive role
(5) how to evaluate a health education programme in terms of its impact on knowledge, attitudes and behaviour
(6) those aspects of daily living likely to be affected by illness or injury; the influence of medical, psychological and social factors in determining the rate of recovery of independence in common conditions; services and professions available to help with rehabilitation after illness or injury and with adaptation to any continuing disability
(7) the duties and responsibilities of doctors and nurses employed in industry and their relationship to the Department of Employment and the Employment Medical Advisory Service.

Students should be able to:

(1) apply the criteria for assessing whether a screening programme for a particular disease is worthwhile
(2) take an occupational history and discuss the value of occupational health records
(3) assess fitness for work and estimate the demands of a particular job; list the major hazards encountered at work and the principles adopted to eliminate or minimize them.

Students should appreciate:

(1) that there may be a conflict between action for the health of the public at large and individual freedom of choice
(2) that nearly all doctor–patient contacts contain some health education
(3) that the purpose of medical rehabilitation is to prevent dependence rather than simply to eliminate disease.

OUTLINE

The aim of preventive medicine is to control disease by intervention, ideally before the disease process has begun but, at least, while it is still amenable to treatment. Prevention depends to a large extent on knowing the natural history of disease – how it begins, how it progresses through the normal to the diseased state and ultimately to recovery, long-term impairment, or death. The ways of discovering the natural history of a disease were outlined in the epidemiology section of Chapter 2. Figure 3.1 shows the stages at which various interventions can occur and this model is helpful in describing the current state of knowledge about any disease and its treatment. Ideally we should be able to quantify not only the incidence rate, but also the proportions of patients in each of the subsequent boxes, because the knowledge is the basis of predicting risk in individuals.

This is possible for virtually all infections and for a few chronic diseases although, in the latter, medical knowledge is not yet sufficiently precise to measure risk, or the probability of a particular outcome, from the combination of factors in any one patient. What can be said, in general terms, is that the ultimate outcome varies with:

(1) the severity of the problem
(2) the success of prevention and treatment
(3) the personal characteristics of the individual.

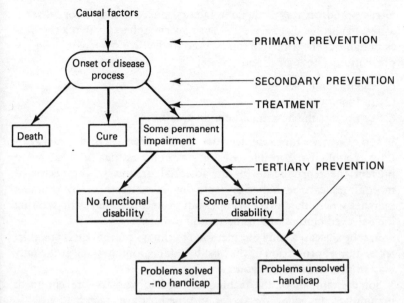

Figure 3.1 Stages of disease and intervention.

There are three stages at which preventive action may be taken:

Primary prevention tries to prevent disease *before* the pathological process has started.

Secondary prevention tries to detect *early* stages of disease, usually presymptomatic, before someone seeks help.

Tertiary prevention actively tries to promote independence by preventing disability as a result of disease. It usually follows acute treatment and includes rehabilitation and routine surveillance to avoid complications.

PRIMARY PREVENTION

One way of regarding disease is as the outcome of a dynamic and ever changing interaction between three entities, namely:

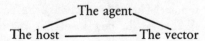

The terms come originally from the epidemiology of communicable diseases and, in these, all three factors must interact before disease arises. In chronic disease we do not know enough to say that a vector is essential, but the principle can be used to devise a strategy of primary prevention. The logical options are:

(1) to eliminate the agent
(2) to block the vector
(3) to protect the host (i.e. the individual).

In some diseases, for example malaria, prevention can be directed at all three. People living in infected areas can take antimalarial tablets to prevent the reproduction of the malarial organism. The vector or mosquitoes can be halted by spraying insecticides or by draining marshes where they breed. People can protect themselves by wearing long-sleeved clothes and using mosquito nets.

In other diseases, only one method of primary prevention is possible; for example, protection of the host by adding iodine to salt is the only way to prevent endemic goitre.

Some examples of the techniques used in primary prevention to manipulate the agent, the vector and the host are given below.

The agent

(1) During the first half of this century it was realized that *bovine tuberculosis* could be communicated to man by drinking infected milk. Organized attempts to eliminate the disease in animals were therefore made, and by *tuberculin testing* and subsequent slaughtering of all infected animals it has been possible to eradicate tuberculosis in milking herds and so control bovine tuberculosis.

(2) Dust fumes and vapours occur in great variety as industrial pollutants and, therefore, it is not surprising that inhalation is the commonest way in which industrial disease is acquired. Some pollutants have an immediate effect while others may have a delayed and prolonged effect such as occurs in *pneumoconiosis*, numerically and socially still an important industrial disease. The introduction of measures such as *dust control in mines* has led to a marked reduction in the incidence of pneumoconiosis in miners. The most effective method of dealing with an industrial hazard is to change the harmful agent for a safe one such as the use of the new insulating materials instead of asbestos.

The vector

Water, which is ingested daily by everyone, may carry pathogenic microorganisms. Thus failure to protect water against contamination is one of the main causes of intestinal infections. It is, therefore, common practice to filter and to *disinfect* water by chlorination before distributing it to consumers. This has been very effective in preventing the transmission of diseases such as the enteric fevers which may be spread by contaminated water.

The host

(1) In the first quarter of this century, *diphtheria* was one of the most frequently fatal diseases of small children. Between 1900 and 1920 the administration of an antitoxin played a large part in reducing the death rate, although the number of cases remained high. However, after active *immunization* of children was introduced in the 1940s the incidence of diphtheria dropped markedly and since protection is now given routinely as part of the primary immunization of children, the disease has virtually been eradicated.

(2) Much evidence has accumulated recently to show that fluoridation of drinking water has a beneficial effect on teeth. Controlled studies have shown a significant reduction in *caries* among children living in areas where the water is fluoridated to a level of one part per million. Nevertheless, there has been considerable opposition to the proposal that there should be general fluoridation of the water supply and it is still a matter for individual local authorities.

Students would find it helpful to apply for themselves the approach of agent–vector–host to other conditions, for example bronchitis, legionnaire's disease or road accidents. The examples detailed above have led to a change in the spectrum of health problems facing us. Infectious disease was formerly a major cause of morbidity and mortality, but successful preventive measures have changed this. As a result, a new set of problems arises, notably those diseases which are associated with an ageing population such as visual and auditory defects and osteoporosis. Changes in attitude and behaviour also lead to different health problems such as those associated with increasing affluence. Third, advances in technology and changes in the physical environment can also lead to changes in the health of a population.

How can we deal with such problems? Is legislation justified or should we concentrate on health education as the most appropriate approach? Where there are a number of possible approaches, the one chosen will obviously vary with the circumstances, for one strategy may be more effective in one situation while others may be more expensive. While it would appear that preventive measures, if proved to be worthwhile, should be applied generally, the key to prevention is frequently the identification of risk factors. People who exhibit one or more of such risk factors will have a greater than average chance of developing the disease and should in times of financial restraint be singled out for preventive measures. In many chronic diseases, such as ischaemic heart disease or cancer, the risk factors are cumulative and thus the highest risk groups are found to have a combination of factors, not all of which may be treatable. However, even to reduce one component of the risk may be worthwhile. It is important to note that this can be done without fully understanding the mechanism by which the disease is produced, i.e. by empirical treatment.

SECONDARY PREVENTION

The principle of secondary prevention is the detection of early, usually presymptomatic, disease to allow earlier treatment which will result in improved outcome. The main technique used is called *screening*, whereby an attempt is made to identify among the apparently healthy those with suspicious or positive findings who must be referred for diagnosis and treatment. Screening has therefore been defined in the following way: the presumptive identification of unrecognized disease or defect by the application of tests, examinations or other procedures which can be applied to differentiate between apparently well persons, who probably have a disease, from those who probably do not.

When a screening test is applied to a whole population it is referred to as *mass screening*. If it is carried out on a selected subgroup regarded as being especially at risk, it is called *selective screening*. With the advent of improved technology and automation, multiple screening tests can be carried out readily for one individual and this is referred to as *multiphasic screening*.

Usually, screening programmes offer tests and people then volunteer to be tested; the implication is that the volunteers will benefit either from early treatment or from reassurance. Sometimes not enough is known about the disease for this commitment to be given, but it is still ethical to include the test in the examination of patients who present with a quite separate problem. This is sometimes called *case-finding*. Even when enough is known to justify a screening programme, case-finding may be considered an acceptable and simpler alternative.

The *criteria* for assessing whether or not it is worthwhile to set up a national screening programme for a disease are:

(1) the disease must be important, e.g. severe, common
(2) the natural history must be known, i.e. the progression from the latent period through early to late pathological processes, including physiological variations
(3) there must be effective treatment for the presymptomatic stage which improves the outcome for the patient
(4) there must be a suitable test or examination – quick, easy, acceptable, economical and reliable (*see below*)
(5) there must be adequate resources for screening and subsequent diagnosis – facilities and staff
(6) consideration must be given as to whether the benefits, of all types, justify the costs involved.

Correct identification of those who have a certain disease and those who do not is of vital importance in this situation, where the health professions are taking the initiative rather than the patient. Screening tests can therefore be defined in specific terms.

Sensitivity and specificity

Sensitivity is defined as the ability of a test to identify correctly those *who actually have the disease* (i.e. to minimize false negatives). Specificity is defined as the ability of a test to identify correctly those *who do not have the disease* (i.e. to minimize false positives).

Reliability

The precision of a test is called the reliability or repeatability of a test. A reliable test will give consistent results when performed more than once on the same individual under the same conditions. The main factors affecting its performance are: variation within the subject, e.g.

physiological variation may occur after meals or through diurnal variation. Variation caused by the observer(s), i.e. differences between different observers (interobserver) or due to variability in the performance of same observer (intraobserver variation). All these variations can be reduced or eliminated by standardization of equipment and procedures and intensive training of observers.

After a screening procedure has been in operation for some time the programme must be evaluated to determine whether it is still achieving its objectives and whether the original justification is still applicable. An example of such a change was found with mass miniature radiography (MMR), which was introduced in 1957 in a national screening programme for pulmonary tuberculosis. By 1970 the incidence rate of the disease had fallen so low that the costs of screening were no longer justified by the numbers of cases picked up and it is now used only when an outbreak is suspected or in selected populations where the risk is higher than usual.

TERTIARY PREVENTION AND REHABILITATION

The concept of actively preventing disability and dependence which might arise as a result of illness or injury may seem very similar to the basis of all treatment. However, there is a difference in the underlying purpose and in the end point. First, you can treat a disease but you can only rehabilitate an individual. Every illness brings with it temporary incapacity or disability, but this can be minimized if there is active anticipation of what is likely to happen and the postacute care that will be required. Hence, the preventive aspect is thinking ahead using knowledge of likely outcomes; it is the early identification of people at risk of disability and the early introduction of means of treating it. Thus it includes a regular surveillance of people with long-term problems, such as hypertension, so that complications may be detected early and, if possible, averted.

For children, the term used is 'habilitation' because the learning of the skills of independence is occurring for the first time, whereas in adults it is a relearning process. Treatment of disease is clearly an integral part of eliminating dependence, but the process of relearning physical, psychological and social functions usually continues for some time after the medical treatment has been completed or stabilized. Thus, while the overall aim of treatment is restoration of normal function, in practice there are different short-term targets. Immediate medical care is geared to eliminating the underlying cause of malfunction, i.e. the disease; rehabilitation is geared to helping the patient out of the 'sick role' back, if possible, to his previous level of independence. It has two phases – preventing disability after illness or injury and promoting adaptation to reduce handicap in those with permanent disability.

For children who are handicapped from birth, there is no previous level of independence to aim for and for them the goal is to close the gap between their independence and that of the average child.

Because everyday living requires many different types of activity, different types of therapy are required in helping people to relearn everyday skills. Rehabilitation as a technique, therefore, involves a varying range of professions who work together to ensure that each patient's particular needs are identified and met. Thus, it requires teamwork as integrated as for working in an operating theatre, but there is often a greater range of variation in the problems being tackled and, sometimes, the most important input is not medical. If this is so, the team must decide who should coordinate the care being given so that the patient is not confused by conflicting advice and there are no gaps or overlaps in therapy. A further difference from the usual function of medicine is that, because independence is the goal, and independence includes being responsible for one's own progress, the relationship with the patient is more one of sharing knowledge and helping him to help himself rather than of doing things to a passive recipient. Such a relationship is time-consuming and requires greater flexibility on the part of the professionals than does clinical medicine, because of the need to take decisions jointly with the patient.

The concept of altering the natural history of a disease or disorder is not strictly applicable in rehabilitation because patients have usually received medical care before the rehabilitation process begins. However, it is possible to describe the outcome after medical care in patients who have and have not been helped to regain independence and, in this way, to identify not only the characteristics of patients who are at high risk of not returning to normal activities, but also the effects of intervention at this stage. An example of a high risk group is heavy goods vehicle licensees (e.g. lorry drivers), who are debarred from such work after a myocardial infarction and require intensive retraining.

In general terms, recovery of independence is related to:

(1) the patient's disease and its expected outcome
(2) social and physical environment
(3) personality and motivation.

Other examples of outcome are:

1 in 5 survivors aged less than 65 does not work again after a myocardial infarction
1 in 2 survivors from head injury with brain damage does return to work
1 in 2 survivors from stroke does regain independence but 1 in 4 has severe disability.

In patients discharged from hospital, high risk factors are:

(1) more than one speciality involved
(2) patient does not know the diagnosis
(3) poor hospital–general practitioner communication
(4) speech or hearing handicap
(5) industrial injuries
(6) previously unemployed.

The treatment of *functional disability* which follows early identification has several crucial components. These are:

(1) *multiprofessional assessment*, initiated usually by the doctor
(2) *social and physical relearning and adaptation*
    (a) daily living
       (i) dressing, washing, toilet, feeding
      (ii) mobility (a) inside the house, (b) outside the house
      (iii) housework, (cooking, cleaning)
    (b) employment, e.g. resettlement, retraining (*see* section on Health at Work, pp. 64–75)
    (c) income
       (i) sickness benefit (for the first 6 months)
      (ii) invalidity benefit and pension (after 6 months)
      (iii) special allowance for the disabled and their families, e.g. constant attendance allowance, mobility allowance, free prescriptions, etc. (*see* Chronically Sick and Disabled Persons Act, 1970)
(3) *continuity of care*, passing on information from hospital to home,

from doctor to other professionals, but always ensuring that someone is coordinating care; regular monitoring to detect early complications in people with long-term problems such as hypertension or diabetes

(4) *patient education* by the primary care team and, for inpatients, in hospital about:
  (a) diagnosis, prognosis, possible effects on life-style
  (b) self-help: how to cope with handicap now and in future (if it remains), the address of a self-help group (if any is working in this field), information about services and benefits
(5) *psychological support* during and after treatment. The most difficult time is usually around 6 months after hospital discharge.

Thus as each patient moves out of the acute phase of an illness every doctor should ask himself or herself the questions in Table 3.1.

Table 3.1 *Preventing dependence: the doctor's check list*

---

(1) Early detection
  do I know the likely outcome of this *disease*?
  what risk factors are present in this *patient*?
(2) Assessment
  what *skills* does this patient have?
  could *other professions* help with assessment or with services?
(3) Practical help
  daily living
  employment
  income
  have I brought in all beneficial services?
  who is coordinating them?
(4) Continuity of care
  who to tell?
  what to tell?
  who is doing the long-term surveillance?
(5) Patient and family education
  what to tell?
  when to tell?
  who to tell?
  who tells?
(6) Motivation and support
  do I understand this patient?
  does the patient understand what is happening?
Is this patient as independent as possible?

Information

Information is the prerequisite for a change in behaviour. A patient can only properly take the drugs prescribed for him if he is informed how so to do. The aims, contents and methods of communicating this information therefore require careful consideration. It is important that the patient understands what the doctor says and that he recalls the advice given. It is well known that up to 50% of advice is forgotten immediately after the consultation, whereas repetition of the information, verbally or in writing, helps the patient to remember more easily (Tones, 1977).

The aims and content of communication have to be considered even more carefully when the message is apparently given to whole populations, such as in campaigns on television, on posters or in newspapers.

The knowledge of what is good for health does not necessarily result in action. For instance, we all know that exercise is important for maintaining physical function; nevertheless, the level of exercise taking in the British community is very low.

Information by itself can create knowledge of what is good or bad for health. That knowledge, however, has to be supported by the wish to act before any behaviour change can follow.

Attitudes

The development of new attitudes in individuals or in society is a complex process. Nevertheless, continuous reinforcement of information can result in changed attitudes. A good example is the change in attitudes towards smoking. Previously, a smoker expected to have the 'right' to smoke whenever he felt like it. Recent opinion surveys, however, show a change; the majority, even of smokers, support restriction of areas where smoking is permissible.

It is also important to remember that health education programmes can have the opposite effect to that which is intended; e.g. in a trial of screening for breast cancer, information intended to encourage women to go for screening created fear to such an extent that it actually prevented women coming forward for screening. Fear, in general, is not a good tool to ensure lasting compliance as it does not affect the underlying values held by the individual. Other negative responses due to fear that individuals cannot cope with are: forgetting that the event has happened (negation) and ridicule. For instance, during World War II when faced with threatening films about syphilis, soldiers did not alter their contact with local prostitutes, but developed jokes about VD.

Therefore, it is advisable to keep in contact with those exposed to health education and attempt to make some estimate of whether the information has had the desired effect. A doctor who gives advice to his patient can question him to ascertain whether the latter has understood and remembers correctly, and can make some assessment as to whether the patient's attitude makes it seem likely that he will comply. Public campaigns in the news media, however, have to be evaluated by public opinion polls before and after the health campaign (or during the campaign if it is of long duration).

The best way to carry out health education varies with the type of message and the types of person it is aimed at. In general, however, it is believed that the group technique is the most effective because it encourages a group of persons with similar problems to ask questions. A group of parents, for instance, can be given information about the nutrition of young children by a dietitian or health education officer and, by discussing among themselves and the health educator the best way to feed young children, they may together develop the motivation to give their children the right balance of a nutritious diet.

Behaviour changes

Positive attitudes towards health do not necessarily result in positive behaviour; for instance, although 85% of drivers in one survey supported the wearing of seat belts, only 17% were actually observed wearing them (Tones, 1977) before it was made compulsory in 1983, when compliance increased markedly to 95%.

Attitudes need a good deal of encouragement to be transformed into action. Parents in the infant feeding group, for instance, not only gained knowledge of infant nutrition and motivation to stick to the rules, but also – by identification with each other and encouragement from the rest of the group – are often pressurized into behaving according to the group norm. This, in fact, is 'peer group pressure' which threatens individuals with becoming outsiders unless they follow the norms of the group in question. It is possible that peer group pressure is so strong that people conform in behaviour without

at first having the attitudes to go with it. The parents in this group
have become a peer group; norms held by this group act as a reference
when parents decide whether or not the feeding behaviour of their
infant is normal. Different peer groups have different norms. Peer
groups can be established for one particular purpose only, such as to
lose weight or to stop gambling. Other health education programmes
make use of existing peer groups, e.g. the 'green cross' education in
schools, or messages for families watching television together (for
instance, a child commenting on Mum's hazardous way of crossing a
street).

Often peer group pressure is enough to give the extra 'push' needed
to change smoking or other habits. Other methods introduce
regulations and/or laws, such as rules to restrict smoking in health
service buildings and laws designed to enforce the wearing of safety
helmets when working on building sites. Both methods reduce the
number of occasions when a person can indulge in his 'undesirable'
behaviour.

The best way to transmit information, to change attitudes and to
encourage specific behaviour depends on which particular action we
want to achieve. In general, discussion groups of interested persons are
seen as most effective (Tones, 1977) because they allow people to
work out their own attitudes and also create peer group pressure
which translates their attitude into action.

As with all inputs into the health services an evaluation by 'before
and after' assessment should be built into any health education
process, whether it is just the transmission of information or an
attempt to modify behaviour.

The measurement of outcome of health education is possible,
provided that the objectives of the programme are specific. For
example: 'my objective as a general practitioner, is to increase from
65% to 80% over the next year the percentage of preschool children
on my list who have completed the immunization schedule'.

Involvement

When considering health education, students are inclined to look to
health education staff and health visitors forgetting that everyone who
has contact with patients can contribute; cumulatively these other
endeavours may well be as important as those of the staff carrying a
full-time responsibility for such services. A useful practical exercise is

to list the various health care professionals who can contribute to health education.

HEALTH EDUCATION

Definition

Health education aims to change behaviour in two separate ways: to prevent self-inflicted disease in people who are exposing themselves to risk, such as smokers; and to promote positive health by adopting habits believed to be health-maintaining, such as balanced diet and exercise. Informing people about 'healthy habits' may be done at individual, local or national level; it can apply to everybody or be directed selectively towards persons especially vulnerable to the particular problem (people 'at risk'). The outcome of a general community approach is much more difficult to assess than individual action; with the former, it is nearly impossible to know who actually received the message or why they responded, whereas doctors or other health workers know clearly which patients they have talked to and by what means they have attempted to influence behaviour. As health education is time-consuming, and therefore expensive, other ways of changing people's behaviour (such as provision of incentives or creation of laws or regulations) have to be taken into consideration before embarking on a major programme. Very often health education is given in conjunction with other, more punitive measures; for instance, advice not to drink and drive is coupled with legislation penalizing those who so do. Less severe, but equally positive, would be the doctor who advises his patient to stop smoking in order to reduce his risk of a further heart attack and who also prohibits smoking in the surgery's waiting room.

Most habits relating to health are acquired during childhood (e.g. attitudes towards pain and illness or dietary habits) and adolescence (e.g. smoking). Hence most behaviour is ingrained and of long standing. If we consider the extended periods of time over which habits have developed, we can appreciate the difficulties faced when setting out to change behaviour.

Health education is a long-term process. Many repeated stimuli are required to produce desired attitudes. However, it is not enough to have the right attitudes – an additional inducement or pressure is needed to change behaviour.

Techniques

Health education has three main components and each step needs reinforcement:

(1) provision of *information*, reinforced by repetition
(2) influencing of *attitudes*, reinforced by learning through personal experience
(3) changes in *behaviour*, reinforced by social situations or environmental circumstances.

ENVIRONMENTAL HEALTH CONTROL

Since the separation of environmental health from general health care in 1974, the community medicine specialists' (community physicians') contribution to environmental health control is confined to giving medical advice on broad policy and planning, and environmental health control is largely the responsibility of the appropriate departments of the local authority. However, although the immediate responsibility no longer lies with community medicine, control of the environment is essential to the maintenance of a healthy way of life. Environmental health control is an extremely wide ranging subject and the following are some of the main aspects:

(1) water supplies
(2) sewage
(3) refuse and industrial waste
(4) food hygiene
(5) port health
(6) air pollution and smoke control
(7) housing standards
(8) noise
(9) nuisances.

Water supplies

In the UK approximately 50 gallons of water per person are used each day and, in recent years, industry has made rapidly increasing demands on our water supplies. The local regional authority is responsible for the quality of water, which must be free from pathogenic and chemical contamination, supplied to households. The water is purified by storage, filtration and finally chlorination and its purity is monitored by routine sampling at various points in the distribution system. The medical adviser at the health authority receives copies of all laboratory reports relating to the public water supply and can initiate whatever action is necessary. Medical advice may also be required regarding, for example, the chlorination of water; the chlorination of the swimming baths; and appropriate screening tests for employees concerned with the public water supply.

Sewage

Sewage is initially treated by breaking it down to small particles and subjecting it to anaerobic bacteria. After 2–3 weeks its bacterial count is reduced by 99% and the remaining sludge can be distributed on the land, in rivers or the sea and it may be chlorinated before final dispersal. The medical officer responsible for environmental health has a duty to advise in certain circumstances where a danger to health may arise as a result of unsatisfactory drainage.

Refuse and industrial waste

An enormous volume of industrial waste is washed into the rivers and seas. While it may be a serious source of bacterial contamination, e.g. from slaughterhouses, on the other hand, laundry water may contain sufficient detergent to eliminate the microflora and fauna of a river. Although industrial wastes are generally resistant to bacterial decomposition, they can be satisfactorily disposed of by the use of expensive refuse treatment plants.

Food hygiene

Food poisoning may be caused by microbes or chemicals. In microbial poisoning the food will either act as the growth medium for the organism or it may be the agent by which it is spread; in chemical poisoning the chemical may be added accidentally or deliberately, as in food preservatives.

Food may become infected at any stage in its production, manufacture, distribution or preparation. As a result strict codes of hygienic practice are promoted and the environmental health officers of the local district authority have the power to inspect all food premises and distribution vehicles to sample foods and to ensure that the standards laid down in the current legislation are met. For those handling food, education in both personal cleanliness and food hygiene as well as in the prevention of contamination and cross-contamination of food is also vital to the prevention of food-borne disease. The environmental health officer also assists the community physician responsible for communicable disease control in the event of an outbreak of food poisoning, both in the investigation of the cause and in instituting the necessary control measures.

Port health (sea and air)

The speed of travelling from abroad has become so great that it is possible for people to enter the UK while incubating infections. Travellers from areas in which important diseases are endemic or epidemic are identified and may be examined. The corresponding community physician in the areas of their destination are notified of their arrival so that surveillance can be continued if necessary.

The hygiene of all ships and aircraft leaving the UK is also supervised as animal and insect vectors of dangerous diseases can be carried. This stems from the danger of ship-borne rats spreading bubonic plague.

In addition, the Environmental Health Department will inspect every consignment of food at its port of entry. If found to be unsatisfactory the food can be prohibited from landing, or the owners may surrender it for destruction. A real danger is that some unscrupulous consignors may bring prohibited food into the country through another port where they have found that the inspection is less strict.

Air pollution and smoke control

Air pollution and smoke control are the responsibility of the local regional authority. Pollutants come mainly from burning of coal and oil and the gases from fuel oil combustion in motor vehicles, which are widely dispersed. It is well known that chest illness is more common in the young and elderly who live in areas with high levels of pollution, and the prevalence of sulphur dioxide and smoke in the environment is measured routinely. If it becomes excessive the regional authority can obtain advice on medical aspects from the appropriate medical officer of the health authority. Authorities may apply to be designated a smoke control area (or 'smokeless zone') which would mean that only smokeless fuels could be used in the home.

Housing standards

District authorities are responsible for the safety and hygiene of domestic dwellings and so have the power to inspect any home after due warning. The Environmental Health Department carries out this task, looking for dampness, inadequate lighting and ventilation, dangerous lack of maintenance and overcrowding. Closure orders can be made when premises are unfit for human habitation.

Overcrowding is much more difficult to deal with as it is not always possible to rehouse a family in a house, or houses, large enough for its needs. In addition, the Environmental Health Department inspects the plans of all proposed buildings and supervises the actual building. An important part of this work is testing the structure and function of the drains.

Noise

Noise or 'unwanted sound' has increased during this century and it is well recognized that employees who spend their working day in high levels of noise eventually become hard of hearing. Damage to hearing can also occur suddenly as the result of sound waves of very high intensity such as occur in explosions, but this is relatively rare. Hearing loss is also part of the ageing process and overall it would appear that modern urban noise may lead to a steady diminution of hearing throughout life. Thus local authorities must concern themselves with sources of noise, e.g. factories, jet engines, discotheques. The Government, in particular, has placed restrictions on aircraft noise at airports, and sonic booms overhead, while checks on the noise produced by heavy road vehicles have been introduced.

Inside factories and all other places of employment it is the employer's responsibility to see that the hearing of his employees is not damaged. Inspectors from the Health and Safety Executive try to ensure that this is carried out.

Nuisances

Nuisances are defined by the Public Health Acts as 'conditions which are prejudicial to health or cause injury, annoyance etc.' Some of the more commonly encountered are defined as 'statutory nuisances', e.g. accumulations of stinking material, and the Environmental Health Department has a duty to require the owner to 'abate the nuisance' or face prosecution.

In contrast, a nuisance may affect only one family which may apply for help from the Environmental Health Department or may have to resort to a private legal action to try to obtain a remedy.

Some statutory nuisances have become offences under recent legislation, e.g. the emission by a factory of dust, fume or vapour into the neighbourhood atmosphere is prohibited under the Health and Saf_ty at Work Act, 1974.

HEALTH AT WORK

Overview

With an accident which actually occurs at work the association with occupation is only too obvious. Exposure to a known poison in the course of work also clearly requires careful supervision and monitoring. Frequently, however, the relationships and the dangers are not obvious and, without a proper medical history, may be missed entirely. For these reasons awareness of a patient's occupation is an essential piece of information in history-taking both for the appropriate care of that individual and for the recognition and prevention of hazards associated with work.

There are two ways in which the majority of doctors are likely to be involved in occupational health problems. First, since something like 80% of all firms in the UK and over 50% of the total work force have no access to doctors or nurses with specialist knowledge of occupational health, their contacts will be through medical examinations, compensation examinations, assessment of fitness to return to work or just the provision of simple advice and reassurance. Therefore, if the medical profession generally is to fulfil these basic roles and be seen to be credible, all doctors must know the basic occupational problems and the basic principles of occupational health to augment their clinical skills.

The second, inevitable, means of involvement in occupational health is through individual patient care, where, as already suggested, there may well be an occupational component in the health problem; students must be able to appreciate and recognize this. This section of the Guide, therefore, has two aims which are to describe:

(1) the nature of occupational health problems and how they are recognized
(2) how these are dealt with and how occupational health problems can be avoided or minimized.

It is appropriate for undergraduate purposes to concentrate on basic principles, to give a method of enquiry and to illustrate these with examples.

The sections which follow merely give examples under the general headings of (a) physical hazards, (b) chemical hazards, (c) occupational respiratory disease, (d) biological hazards and, finally, (e) recognition and control. Detailed notes can be found in the further reading suggestions at the end of the chapter.

As already indicated, the dangers of working in steel-making or on oil rigs are immediately obvious; the dangers of working with radioactivity or asbestos have also become obvious but, unfortunately, only after the relevant substances had been in use for some considerable time. Complete protection of a worker is extremely difficult and two somewhat conflicting factors are involved. The first is the tendency to believe that a degree of risk (and thereby a proportion of casualties) at work is inevitable, a view surprisingly often held by employees themselves. The other element is a tendency to balance economic and toxic considerations against each other – a view not surprisingly held by some employers.

There is, therefore, a two-way conflict between what society would like and what it is willing to pay. As in all matters, standards are relative to what is acceptable at any point of time.

(1) Society endorses something because it does not know a hazard exists.
(2) Society endorses the hazard because it cannot afford to make it safe in the short-term, or even worse, because it cannot see an alternative and is not willing to do without the product.

In the latter situation, society solves the problem (or salves its conscience) by paying people a lot of money to do a dangerous job or paying them generous compensation if they get hurt. Some employees indeed foster this approach and society also condones it:

The more spent on making a job safe, the less appropriate is 'danger' money and some people are often only too willing to take risks for reward.

The more spent on making a job safe the more it costs and society is at times quite willing to pay others to take risks for the general benefit.

The only factor that changes (and then only slowly) is the level of risk that society finally sees as unacceptable at any price – the problem is not the principle itself, but the point at which the principle is applied. The medical profession has a duty to persuade and ensure that these levels match the current state of knowledge and do not lag behind. The lists that follow briefly summarize examples of that current knowledge.

Physical hazards

Nature	*Result*	*Comment*
Injury	Cuts, burns, foreign bodies, fractures	Guards, automatic switches, fail safe locks and good housekeeping
Posture	Arthritis	Straight back lifting
	Backache	Ergonomics
Vibration	Dead hand	Pneumatic hammers,
	White finger	Chain saws
	Joint degeneration	
Heat	Heat exhaustion	Only a few special industries in the UK
Cold	Cold exhaustion	More common especially offshore, hill walking, cold store – prevention best, but know treatment
High pressure	Decompression sickness	Divers – know the symptoms and treatment

Light	Infra-red: cataract and microwave	Automation and shields
	Ultraviolet: burns and cataract	Welders, proper protection for
	Laser: retinal burns	eyes, reflection at a distance
Ionizing radiation	Somatic: cancer, leukaemia	Protect individual and record
	Genetic abnormalities	cumulative exposure
Electricity	Cardiac arrest	Know resuscitation procedures and arrange training in these for relevant personnel
Noise	Deafness (gradual onset)	Redesign equipment, baffles and earmuffs

Accident or injury prevention is nearly always commonsense and most solutions are obvious given some thought; to help with this a time-honoured set of steps can be followed.

Substitution: mechanical fork lift instead of manual lifting; if visibility over a load is poor, drive fork lift in reverse; if physical hazard, replace people with machines; if mechanical hazard, substitute a safer tool.

Automation: this is taking machine replacement a stage further (i.e. no operator or a remote operator).

Enclosure: obvious technique – guards/fences/barriers. Ideally enclose whole job with operator outside (radioactivity/microwaves/lasers/noise/dust, suppression by water/sand blasting etc.

Local exhaust ventilation and general ventilation: carry away as quickly as possible any hazardous material (mostly with gas and dust) or, duct in cold air (where excess heat is the problem).

Up to this point most of these measures are not under the control of the worker. If it becomes necessary to rely on a worker, control is less certain (e.g. a machine should switch off automatically if a guard is moved, rather than switching it off separately before removing a guard).

Protection of the worker: although protective clothing, goggles, aprons, respirators, visors, ear muffs, are all of value (as are good washing facilities), these should be considered as secondary to the other actions listed above.

Education of employer and employee: if a risk exists, both employer and employee should be aware of it. It should not be minimized. Explain the precautions even if it means stating the obvious.

Chemical hazards

Nature	*Agent*	*Result*
Solids	Fibreglass	Dermatitis
	Phenol	Toxic if absorbed
Vapours and gases	Carbon dioxide	Asphyxia if in a sufficient concentration
	Carbon monoxide, hydrocyanide	Toxic even in low concentrations
	Chlorine, ammonia	Irritant and lethal if concentration high
	Aromatic hydrocarbons	Mostly organic and very toxic if inhaled – damaging liver, kidney, brain and blood-forming organs
Liquids and droplets	Chromic acid	Perforated nasal septum and carcinoma of lung
	Oils	Dermatitis and cancer
	Caustics	Tissue destruction
	Glues	Dermatitis
	Tetraethyl lead	Poisoning (as with gases)
	Organic phosphorus	Pulmonary oedema, muscular weakness

Metallic and non-metallic dusts	Lead	General poisoning
	Mercury	Liver, kidneys, nervous tissue
	Beryllium	Sarcoidosis
	Asbestos	Asbestosis, bronchitis
	Silica	Pneumoconiosis

The preventive principles are the same (substitution/enclosure/protection etc.), but the techniques are different. Environmental and personnel monitoring is also necessary, as is the setting of safe limits estimated by clinical and biological measures. Sometimes the work is so dangerous there is a requirement to work in teams with each member checking on the others. These are often laid down by codes of practice and the actions needed in an emergency are routinely rehearsed.

Occupational respiratory disease

Nature	*Agent*	*Result*
Allergy	After years of exposure to wood dust or printers' gum	Late onset asthma
Carcinogenesis	Wood dust	Cancer of nasal passages
	Uranium, nickel	Lung and bronchus
	Asbestos	Pleura
Chemicals	Ammonia, phosphorus	Irritation and oedema
Infection	Classic example	Anthrax
	Hazards of health workers	Tuberculosis
	Suggested by occupation or hobby	Psittacosis
Fibrosis benign	Iron	Siderosis
	Tin	Stannosis

disabling	Silica	Silicosis
	Asbestos	Asbestosis
	Coal	Pneumoconiosis
Chronic bronchitis	Dust	
	Atmospheric pollution	
	Cement	

Biological hazards

Agent	*Result*
Bacteria and viruses	Infection may enter any wound causing sepsis or tetanus
	Many diseases may be contracted from animals or animal products e.g. brucellosis, leptospirosis, anthrax, erysipeloid
Fungi and moulds	Farmer's lung, byssinosis actinomycosis, ringworm
Internal and external parasites	Worms and flukes in animal handlers, miners and tunnel .vorkers
Vegetable material	Dermatitis and allergic reactions. Certain wood dusts – cancer of the nasal sinuses.

A need for detailed knowledge of particular hazards or industries will ultimately depend upon the part of the country in which the doctor practises but, common to all, is the responsibility to find out *all* the occupations (not just the present one) the patient has had; in many cases it will be the only clue to what is wrong.

Recognition and control

In the middle of the nineteenth century the earliest attempts to improve working conditions placed greatest emphasis on controlling the previously excessive number of hours worked and on prohibiting certain types of work for women and children, e.g. handling lead. These deserved their priority, but since then an enormous amount of legislation has been enacted in an attempt to control the working environment, all made necessary by progressive changes in the nature of work and improvements in our understanding of its effects on health. So much so that by 1974 it could be said that the only occupation involving a significant number of people and not controlled by statute or regulation was domestic service.

Prior to 1974, legislation provided the framework for the control of specific working environments by designating responsibility to particular departments of government, making various restrictions and prohibitions, permitting the appropriate minister to make regulations to extend the controls, and by setting up an inspectorate for their enforcement. However, too many agencies were involved and apathy and ignorance at all levels in industry, together with financial pressures, tended to limit their effectiveness in preventing ill health. Therefore, a change in legislative emphasis was introduced by the Health and Safety at Work etc. Act, 1974. The new approach attempts to overcome these problems by involving people at all levels of responsibility in specified tasks, each aimed at improving the healthiness and safety of the working environment. For example, management is required to prepare and revise when necessary a written statement of its health and safety policy and the organization and arrangements for its execution. This policy must be shown to all employees, who must also be informed, trained and supervised so far as is reasonable and practicable to ensure their health and safety at work. In addition, safety representatives must be appointed from among the employees, either by trade unions or by election and they must be consulted by management with a view to promoting health and safety as a cooperative effort.

These matters cannot be left solely to the employers and employees and so an outside independent group is needed to lay down standards and see that they are observed. In the UK this is carried out by the Health and Safety Commission and their policies are implemented by a separate executive. Because there is a practical limit to the amount of supervision possible, control is concentrated on the inspection of the most dangerous occupations and the detection and identification of so far unrecognized hazards.

The Act is intended to change attitudes. It does not replace, and instead consolidates, the long list of statutes controlling the various working environments, but it does reorganize the supervision and brings it all under one department.

The Act introduces the concept of 'the code of practice' (*see* p. 69) which is meant to provide a means of plugging any gaps in the law, by giving practical guidance to the requirements of the Act and any other statutory provisions. These Codes of Practice which are issued by the Health and Safety Commission have a curious position in law because they are not enforceable, yet failure to observe their provisions can be used as evidence of a contravention of a statutory requirement or prohibition in any relevant enactment.

The Health and Safety at Work etc. Act provides two other major monitors – the control of 'emissions into the atmosphere of noxious or offensive substances from prescribed classes of premises', and 'the transport by road, storage and handling of dangerous substances'.

In the statutes affecting the working environment the first provisions deal in general terms with health by, for example, requirements for cleanliness, ventilation and control of temperature; with safety by, for example, requirements that moving machinery be guarded, cranes and lifts be tested for their safe working load and that specified fire precautions be taken; and with welfare by, for example, requiring the provision of drinking water and facilities for washing and rendering first-aid.

Formal industrial health supervision falls into two groups:

(1) *occupational health services*: doctors, nurses and laboratories provided and wholly paid for by the employer. Currently these cover about one-third of the work force in this country.
(2) the Government service of the *Employment Medical Advisory Service* providing supervision and advice, but not treatment. For obvious reasons part of this supervision covers firms with their own occupational health services, but in practice most time is spent with firms not having such services.

There is no general requirement for industry to provide a medical or nursing service for itself, except first-aid training for those in charge. However, various acts empower the appropriate ministers to require specific industries to provide medical services, examples being British Rail and the Atomic Energy Authority. Accidents at work causing loss of 3 or more days of work and the diseases listed in the Act or in regulations (*see* p. 37) must be notified to HM Chief Inspector of Factories as soon as possible. If such a disease has not been notified already, any doctor attending such a patient is required to notify it, the purpose being the prevention of further injury or illness. The Factory Inspector and, where appropriate, the Employment Medical Adviser will investigate the situation and make recommendations. When the problem is technically complex, inspectors who specialize in chemical, electrical or engineering matters are consulted.

The matching of the capabilities of the industrial juvenile to the demands of a particular job is the responsibility of the *Youth Employment Service*, advised by the school medical officer and the employment medical adviser.

In practice, the school medical officer notifies the employment medical adviser of every school-leaver who has a defect which may affect his fitness for unrestricted employment. The employment medical adviser, a doctor with training and experience in occupational medicine and employed by the Department of Employment, examines the teenager and may prohibit him from taking up certain jobs. The intention is to try to ensure that young people with impaired health do not have their condition made worse by the demands of the job (e.g. asthma in a dusty atmosphere), but it avoids the situation where every young person has to have a medical examination for each new job, as was the requirement until 1974.

The employment medical adviser is also responsible for the medical supervision of people employed in 'dangerous trades'. These are named in regulations and the intervals between the examinations are specified. The intention is to detect at the earliest possible moment signs of the absorption of some toxic substance before any serious harm has been done. At the same time, the inspector will try to find out how the normal protective routine has failed and allowed this absorption. Where an industry has its own medical advisers (often referred to as factory doctors), they may be permitted by the Minister of Employment to supervise the health of employees in dangerous trades.

Should an environmental hazard be suspected which requires investigation with special equipment, the Department of Employment can deploy mobile laboratories. In addition, there are a few private occupational hygiene laboratories offering a service to industry and large companies usually have their own.

Prescribed diseases

There is a list of occupational diseases which are considered preventable and a worker who contracts one of them may receive compensation under the industrial injuries scheme. 'Occupational asthma', for example, is the most recent addition to the list, which is given in Waldron (1979, Appendix 2).

Occupational rehabilitation

The Disabled Persons (Employment) Acts, 1944 and 1958 were passed to try to alleviate the difficulties that some disabled people have in obtaining and keeping suitable employment. They aim to help all the disabled whether physical or mental, congenital or acquired (*see* also pp. 52–5). The Department of Employment maintains a register of people who are likely to be disabled for at least 6 months. Registration is voluntary and the disabled person must apply for admission to the register. Medical assessment is usually required. Many disabled persons decline to apply for registration as they believe that to publicize their disabilities in this way reduces rather than increases their employment opportunities. The Acts require that every employer of more than 20 people must employ a quota of registered disabled people. The quota is fixed at 3% at present.

Under the Acts, the Department of Employment has set up employment rehabilitation centres (ERC) in the main industrial areas. These provide suitable work experience for people requiring a gradual adjustment to working conditions after injury or serious illness. An important part of their function is to assess the patient's capabilities and with this knowledge to suggest suitable occupations. The courses last 8–12 weeks, but do not train members for new jobs. For this purpose the Acts establish skill centres and authorize individuals to attend there or local technical colleges, whichever is the more appropriate to the need of the individual.

So that the most seriously handicapped, still employable, persons should have a chance of work, the Minister is empowered to 'designate employment' as available solely to the disabled. To date only car-park attendants and lift operators have been designated in this way. To the same end, the Acts authorize the establishment of sheltered workshops in which the disabled can work at their own speed and still earn a living. The job is not necessarily simple or trivial, but both worker and management are free from the pressures of commercial competition and the need to make a profit. Remploy Ltd. is the main example, with over 90 factories of various kinds throughout Britain some of which provide work at home for those unable to reach a factory.

All major local authorities were required to arrange for sheltered employment in workshops for the blind, but as the prevalence of blindness has fallen many authorities have extended the facility to people with other handicaps, including mental subnormality, again providing work at home, where necessary, for the housebound. In addition, there are many sheltered workshops run by charitable organizations, but these are usually intended for a particular type of disability, e.g. for disabled ex-servicemen or for people disabled by tuberculosis.

To carry out the provisions of the Acts at local level the Department of Employment has disablement resettlement officers (DROs) to liaise with employers, the social services and the medical profession. These officers also work in employment rehabilitation centres with psychologists, instructors and doctors.

Summary

The aims of the legislation and the main ways of exercising control are summarized in Table 3.2.

Table 3.2 *Central control (Health and Safety at Work Act, 1974)*

Aims of the Act
  to secure health, safety and welfare of workers
  to protect others from risks from works (including pollution of environment)
  to control dangerous substances and activities

Means of control
  Health and Safety Executive (1000 inspectors)
  employment medical advisory service (100 specialists)
  responsibility on employers
  involvement of trade unions
  responsibility on employees
  notifiable diseases and '3 day' accidents
  codes of practice or regulations
  prescribed diseases

Finally, if faced with a health problem at work go back to the basic principles detailed on p. 67 and, in individual cases of illness, never forget the prime rule always to obtain a full occupational history.

INTERNATIONAL HEALTH ORGANIZATIONS

History

International collaboration over health matters began in 1851 when the first international meeting was held in Paris, the concern being with the control of epidemic diseases. In 1907 an International Office of Public Health was set up in Paris to deal with quarantine restrictions. It lasted for 40 years and was absorbed into the World Health Organization in 1947. In 1921 another health organization was set up within the League of Nations and it undertook to obtain international agreement about classification of disease and causes of death. It also fostered the idea of expert committees, with international representation, thereby strengthening international collaboration. Both ceased to function during the Second World War and their functions were assumed by the United Nations Relief and Rehabilitation Administration (UNRRA). After the war, the desirability of having a neutral international body to govern world health policy was recognized and, under the auspices of the Charter of the United Nations, the World Health Organization (WHO) came into being. The WHO is by far the largest international health organization; some other international organizations with their functions are summarized below.

(1) Other governmental agencies, e.g. UNICEF (United Nations International Children's Emergency Fund) predominantly concerned with child welfare and FAO (Food and Agriculture Organization) concerned with nutrition
(2) Non-governmental agencies, e.g. International Union Against Tuberculosis
(3) Red Cross agencies, particularly active in wartime and in civil disasters
(4) Universities and research institutes, international collaboration achieved by visiting and seconding staff to work away from home usually to gain experience in a particular speciality
(5) Religious missions, a particular contribution to the treatment of leprosy.

The WHO definition of health: health is a state of complete physical, mental and social well-being and not merely the absence of disease or infirmity.

The WHO administration

The WHO meets annually. Each member state sends three delegates to the Annual Assembly which is held in Geneva and meets for 3 weeks. The assembly defines policy, approves the budget and reviews the work done. An executive board consisting of 24 members, eight of whom retire annually, meets twice each year and executes the policy. The Director-General with the aid of five Assistant Directors-General is responsible for the Secretariat and the various aspects of international health, e.g. communicable disease control, epidemic intelligence, pharmacology and toxicology. The world is also subdivided into six regions, the administration being the responsibility of a regional director and regional committee. The headquarters for America is in Washington, USA, for Africa in Brazzaville, Congo, for the Eastern Mediterranean in Alexandria, Egypt, for Europe in Copenhagen, Denmark, for South-East Asia in New Delhi, India and for the Western Pacific in Manila, Philippines.

The work of the WHO

At international level

Epidemic intelligence. Under the International Sanitary Regulations governments are obliged to inform the WHO of the occurrences of the quarantinable diseases. The Regulations are revised annually and amended as necessary. The organization is also responsible for disseminating information about 'epidemic' diseases worldwide in its *Weekly Epidemiological Record*.

Communicable disease control. In 1958, the WHO assembly unanimously adopted a resolution initiating a worldwide programme for eradication of smallpox providing, for example, teams of experts to work out eradication programmes and also technical advice on the production of freeze-dried vaccines. The global eradication of smallpox was announced on 8 May, 1980. However, recently (1986) it has been shown that the virus can remain viable in dried form, e.g. in corpses, for indefinite periods.

Biological standardization. International biological standards and reference preparations are established by the WHO and distributed free of charge to national laboratories.

Health statistics and classification of diseases. The WHO has been responsible for the development of definitions and classification of disease which facilitate international comparison of morbidity and mortality patterns. In 1966, the WHO assembly emphasized the necessity of reliable statistics for health planning and effective operation of services.

Non-communicable disease control. Non-communicable diseases have, in recent years, reached epidemic proportions and the WHO has paid particular attention to various problems as they relate to cardiovascular disease, cancer, dental health, mental health, nutrition, smoking and drug abuse.

Health care. In 1978, an International Conference on Primary Health Care, sponsored by the WHO and UNICEF, was held at Alma Ata in the USSR and generated the Declaration of Alma Ata. This sets a goal of *Health for All by the Year 2000* and states that primary health care is the key to attaining this target as part of normal social and economic development. Since then the WHO has created two formal groups – one on Global Health Development and the second on Health 2000 Resources. The underlying principle reverses previous WHO practice in that the aim is to promote the growth of health-giving activities by and within small populations rather than to hand out services from the centre. Much of the work of the WHO has now been redirected to this goal. It is often wrongly assumed that these goals are only meant for underdeveloped or Third World countries, but reference to the Black Report (1980) on health inequalities in the UK quickly shows that such topics have still not been met in countries with relatively sophisticated health systems.

At national level

Specific national projects. The WHO is willing to give assistance to any member state whose government requests help and is prepared to cooperate actively on a specific project.

Malaria eradication. The WHO is advising many countries on the optimum methods of spraying insecticides to eradicate the mosquito which carries malaria and also advises on the treatment of those who have already contracted the disease. Some 57% of the population of the originally malarious areas have now been freed from the disease, but there are still in excess of 350 million people in the world exposed to malaria without the protection offered by eradication schemes.

Clear drinking water and sanitation. Some 200 million people have no clean drinking water and one out of every four hospital beds in the world is occupied by a patient who is ill because of polluted water. While the WHO does not do any actual construction work, it assists countries with the complex legal, financial, engineering and administrative problems of water supply development. The WHO has also been active in educating sanitary engineers particularly for developing countries.

Organization of health services. The WHO gives advice on national and local health planning and may also act in an advisory capacity in states of emergency. It has taken particular interest in the planning of laboratory services, occupational health problems and maternal and child health and is now promoting local, primary health care within all member nations, whatever their state of economic development.

The work of the WHO in education and research

One of the main obstacles to improving world health is the shortage of doctors, nurses and other health workers. The WHO has, therefore, devoted considerable resources to the education and training of health workers and also to establishing new medical schools. The WHO is also active in postgraduate education and has a scheme whereby fellowships are granted to qualified health workers who usually go abroad to learn new techniques before setting up a service in their own country.

The WHO supports research in many fields, notably cardiovascular disease, neoplastic diseases and mental health and has an important role as a coordinator of research projects. To this end the WHO convenes international meetings and provides grants for research purposes.

The main concerns of the WHO in the regions are summarized below.

Africa
communicable disease control
water supplies and sanitation

America
education and research
organization of health services

SE Asia
communicable disease control
malaria eradication
water supplies and sanitation

Europe
non-communicable disease
health care planning

Eastern Mediterranean
malaria eradication
communicable disease control

Western Pacific
non-communicable disease control
organization of health service

FURTHER READING

Health education
Tones B. (1977) *Effectiveness and Efficiency in Health Education*, pp.
   12–14; 40–4. Edinburgh: Scottish Health Education Unit

Health at work
Waldron H. A. (1979) *Lecture Notes and Occupational Medicine*.
   Oxford: Blackwell
Trades Union Congress. (1979) *Safety and Health at Work*. London:
   TUC

Prevention – general
Department of Health and Social Security. (1976) *Prevention and
   Health: Everybody's Business*, pp. 31–71. London: HMSO
Morris J. (1975) Four cheers for prevention. In: *Uses of Epidemiol-
   ogy*. Edinburgh: Churchill Livingstone

Prevention of particular problems
Scottish Home and Health Department. (1981) *Slainte Mhath (good*

health). The Medical Problems of Excessive Drinking. London: HMSO

Department of Health and Social Security. (1978) *Prevention and Health: Eating for Health.* London: HMSO

Department of Health and Social Security. (1978) *Reducing the Risk: Safer Pregnancy and Childhood.* London: HMSO

Department of Health and Social Security. (1980) Inequalities in Health. Report of a working group chaired by Sir Douglas Black. London: HMSO

Department of Health and Social Security. (1981) *Prevention and Health: Avoiding Heart Attacks.* London: HMSO

Rehabilitation

Blaxter M. (1977) *The Meaning of Disability*, pp. 18–37; 56–88; 220–37. London: Heinemann Medical

Chapter

4

Medical and Social Care

THE AIMS AND PRIORITIES OF HEALTH SERVICES • TYPES OF CARE •
PROFESSIONS IN HEALTH CARE • LOCAL AUTHORITY SERVICES •
VOLUNTARY AGENCIES • SERVICES FOR CHILDREN AND OLD
PEOPLE • RESOURCES, CHOICES AND DECISION-MAKING • SOCIAL
SECURITY • INTERNATIONAL HEALTH CARE SYSTEMS

This chapter outlines the professions and services with which doctors
work for the benefit of their patients. It starts with a comment on the
aims of the UK National Health Service so that students have some
idea of its current problems and achievements.

OBJECTIVES

Students should know:

(1) the broad organization of health and social services in the UK and
    how this differs in other countries; the major medical problems of
    less well developed countries and how they may be affected by
    social change
(2) how local hospitals, primary care, community care and social
    services are organized and interrelated
(3) who is responsible for occupational and environmental health
    services and how they are coordinated with general health care
(4) the contribution of the other professions involved in health and
    social care; the after-care services that exist and which groups of
    patients are most likely to need them
(5) current views on the achievements and failures of the health
    services in the UK and ideas about future services
(6) why choices always have to be made of what care to provide, and
    some of the techniques and information involved in ranking
    priorities for care

(7) the way in which the public and professionals can contribute to the planning and running of the health service
(8) why the proportion of older people is increasing throughout the world, the implications for welfare services of all types and the impact on disease patterns and medical services in particular.

THE AIMS AND PRIORITIES OF HEALTH SERVICES IN THE UK

There has always been a public responsibility for health; even before the causes of infection were understood, quarantine and isolation existed. However, apart from these obvious public actions, medical care for the paramount problem of infections was haphazard and covered only those patients who by choice or opportunity happened to go to a doctor. Unfortunately, infectious disease could not be controlled just by some people seeking medical advice, because the basic need was not simply to treat people who were sick, but also to change the behaviour of people before they became ill. This still applies, as it also does in chronic disease.

The original health service planned in the late 1930s was based on society's experience of poverty and infectious disease, and it was not appreciated during the planning (perhaps in part because of the upheaval of the Second World War) that the action on sanitation, education and housing initiated many years before had taken effect. Ironically, the health service was therefore designed for a problem which had already been solved and not for the new challenges which were beginning to emerge. Over the last 30 years there has been a complete change in the pattern of disease, and today the major problems are chronic, multiple disorders with intermittent acute episodes. Added to this is the fact that we have an increasingly aged population with a greater proportion of chronic sick, i.e. more old people with major or multiple and incapacitating disabilities. Events have overtaken us. For obvious reasons, we are most aware of acute illness and there is a danger that we have allowed some of our other services to fall below what society considers an acceptable minimum.

Twenty years ago, when Kenneth Robinson was Minister of Health he said that the aim of the NHS was to provide all the services required by individuals at different stages of their lives either singly or in combination. At present, it would be fair to say that the services needed by people who are disabled rather than acutely ill are not being

provided in anything like the quantity that is required. When the
health service started there were so many deficiencies that vast
additional resources had to be provided, with the result that those
services capable of using the money immediately grew faster. In this
way the individual services developed their own separate momentum
and grew in terms of what they were technically capable of achieving
for the patients they saw, rather than of what was actually needed by
the people they never saw. The public began to think that it was
becoming possible to eliminate illness by new techniques and that the
more money that went into the new acute services, the quicker this
would happen. When Sir Keith Joseph was Minister of Health he said:
'This is a very fine country in which to be acutely ill or injured, but
take my advice and do not become old or frail or mentally ill here'.
That was said in 1973 and the health service today still has three
major problems.

(1) There are inequalities in the distribution of health services across
    the UK
(2) The services required for caring for disabled people do not always
    match up to the current image of what medical services in a highly
    technical society should be doing, i.e. they are not viewed as a
    'medical need' or even, by some, as a responsibility of the health
    service. As a result, there is a limit to the number of people willing
    to undertake such work in the health service and very few
    institutional places which provide simple nursing care
(3) Given that resources in terms of money and people are not
    unlimited, how are the priorities to be rearranged? Choices have to
    be made, such as between providing simple help for people who
    cannot feed themselves or go to the toilet unaided, and providing
    operations for men who want vasectomy. Against this back-
    ground, in 1976 and 1977, the Government issued the following
    statements on two major policy issues:

    (a) *Prevention and Health* (1977) Cmnd. 7047 HMSO, which
        followed a discussion document, *Prevention and Health:
        Everybody's Business* (1976)
    (b) *Priorities in the Health and Social Services: The Way Forward*
        (1977) HMSO, and *Health Services in Scotland: The Way
        Ahead* (1976) HMSO

These are likely to continue to influence the direction of health services for the next decade at least and, therefore, the context in which clinical care is delivered.

As well as a move towards prevention, the papers propose a shift of resources from the acute sector to services for the chronically sick and handicapped and from hospital to community care. The priority groups identified in these reports are elderly people, mentally ill people, mentally handicapped people and those with physical or sensory handicap. The priority services in England and Wales (other than prevention) were maternity, primary care and services for children at risk while, in Scotland, they were services for multiply deprived families.

Associated with these are two other shifts in emphasis on the manner in which health and illness should be handled. One is the philosophy expressed in *Prevention and Health: Everybody's Business*, namely, that everyone in society should be aware of their responsibility for promoting their own well-being. This approach is also integral to the policy of the WHO, referred to in Chapter 3, and is likely to be a major influence on the role of doctors and health services in the future.

The second shift of emphasis concerns the balance between different professions and agencies who help ill people (*see* Table 4.1, p. 89). The number of specialized technicians who are part of teams providing acute care (such as renal dialysis) has grown in recent years. As well as this, the increasing proportion of problems which require long-term help, supervision and support has led to greater involvement of professions with skills which doctors, as they are now trained, do not have. For example, comprehensive care of children should ensure that physical handicap does not create secondary handicaps by debarring such children from normal schooling. Helping people to return to work (including housework) brings in the specialized services of occupational therapists and of the employment medical advisory service. In older people, the aim is to promote and maintain their ability to function as full members of a community (if they so wish); this may require not only physical help, but also the services of social work and voluntary groups to facilitate mobility and human contact for the high proportion who live alone and have no family. There is thus an increasing emphasis in all aspects of care on the contribution of professions other than doctors. The need to coordinate their work was discussed in Chapter 3 (Rehabilitation) and an outline of their roles and skills is included in this Chapter. It is also interesting and useful to compare the balance of services and professions in different countries and some examples are itemized in Table 4.2 (p. 123).

These changes in balance and direction of services have occurred in response to the changing health problems which have been outlined. However, the overall aims of the health service remain as originally devised; these were summarized by the Royal Commission on the National Health Service (1979):

'We believe the NHS should:

* encourage and assist individuals to remain healthy
* provide a broad range of services of a high standard
* provide equality of access to these services
* provide a service free at the time of use
* satisfy the reasonable expectations of its users
* remain a national service responsive to local needs.'

It will be clear by now that achieving these laudable aims must be a matter of compromise because, with finite resources, they are inevitably in competition. For example 'equality of access' and a 'broad range of services of a high standard' may require some national centralization of services and hence reduce local access for some to achieve general access for all. Also, there are still wide variations in rates of resources provided in different areas or regions. By the RAWP and SHARE reports (*see* p. 124) resources are allocated according to a formula which allows for differences in mortality experience (SMR), age composition of the population and the known pattern of previous use of services. (It also allows for 'cross boundary flow' of patients to national services and the special responsibilities for teaching hospitals.) The redistribution, which will be spread over 10 years means, for example, that the health services each year in one authority will receive about 2% less of the total monies for health, while another will receive 2% more. This may seem a small shift but, ultimately, it will represent a reduction for the loser of 16% of its 1976 allocation and an increase for the gainer of nearly 40% (in real terms). Obviously, when the increase in total funding available to the health service is minimal or non-existent, then any reduction imposed under these schemes will cause difficulties in maintaining the level of service in those areas affected.

However, even though RAWP and SHARE attempt to even out

distribution *between* health authorities, differences *within* areas are the responsibility of health authorities. There is a great deal of evidence (e.g. Black Report, 1980, on *Inequalities in Health*), not only that there are different rates of provision within areas, but also that there are fewer services in locations with higher levels of need as judged by infant mortality rates. Thus not all the aims have been attained in full, but gradually the range, location and quality of services are being extended.

TYPES OF CARE

As has been stated, the money to provide health services comes from the government. Despite the intention to shift care away from the acute hospital services, the proportion of expenditure on non-hospital services is slow to change. Figure 4.1 shows the sources and uses of money, including the part provided and used by local government in the social work or 'personal social' services (*see* pp. 98 and 102). The government allocates to health a proportion of the money which it has at its disposal from general taxation, and this is the main source. The health service competes with other public services such as education and defence for a share of these exchequer funds. Contrary to popular belief, less than 10% comes from weekly National Insurance contributions.

The main expenditure is on the hospital and specialist services. Note that the pharmaceutical costs (of about £1000 million in 1979/80) are only for drugs prescribed in general practice and exceed the cost of the general medical practitioners themselves. The latter take up only 5% of the total expenditure, although about one-half of the doctors in the UK work in general practice. Overall, staff account for about three-quarters of the money spent each year and Table 4.1 shows the numbers and types of staff who work in the health service.

The services and staff outlined in Table 4.1 are described later in this Chapter but, before considering how they are organized in detail, it is helpful to have an idea of the types of care they and others give to patients or people with health-related problems. At this stage, the concept of care becomes much wider than the provision of services by the government. It includes all the illnesses which people treat themselves, and the help which family members and friends give each other for acute or long-term illnesses. Such care is less easy to measure because it is not formalized, but there is enough knowledge from

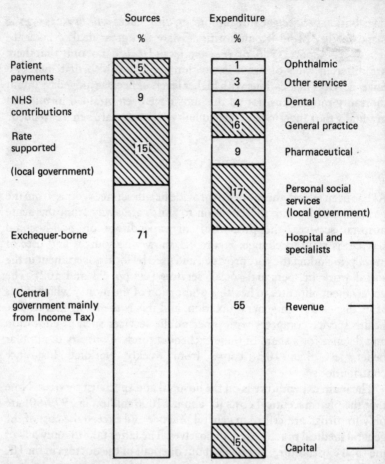

Figure 4.1 Health and personal social service finance, Great Britain. Although the total changes each year, the percentage distribution within sources of money and within expenditure is fairly constant. (From DHSS, 1986 *Health and Social Services for England with Summary Tables for Great Britain 1985*. London: HMSO.)

surveys and other special studies to say that for about three-quarters of the episodes of illness that occur in a year, medical help is not sought. Thus it is possible to outline the approximate distribution of types of illness and 'care' in the UK today. Figure 4.2 shows this in the form of an iceberg, with the problems which patients bring to a doctor above the water-line and the others below the surface.

Table 4.1 *Manpower in the health and personal social services[1] in the UK (thousands)*

	1976	1978	1979	1980	1981
Regional and area health authorities[2] medical and dental[3]	41.7	43.9	45.3	46.5	47.4
nursing and midwifery (excluding agency staff)	429.6	440.1	449.2	466.1	492.8
professional and technical (excluding works)	65.4	70.8	74.1	76.4	80.2
administrative and clerical	116.6	119.1	121.8	124.7	129.1
other staff (including ancillary, works, maintenance, and ambulance)	272.4	273.4	272.4	274.4	276.1
Total regional and area health authorities	925.6	947.2	962.8	988.1	1025.6
Family practitioner services general medical practitioners	27.1	28.0	28.5	29.2	30.1
general dental practitioners	13.6	14.1	14.4	14.7	15.2
ophthalmic medical practitioners, ophthalmic opticians and dispensing opticians	7.9	8.1	8.4	8.9	9.0
Total family practitioner professionals	48.7	50.2	51.3	52.8	54.3
Dental estimates board and prescription pricing authority/ prescription pricing division[4]	4.4	4.5	4.6	4.8	4.7
Personal social services	228.2	238.3	242.4	249.4	250.9

[1] Figures for family practitioner services are numbers; all other figures are whole-time equivalents. The total of health authorities' staff and family practitioners contains an element of duplication since some practitioners have been counted under more than one of the categories shown. The figures relate as closely as possible to 30 September. Figures for Northern Ireland refer to 31 December, except for the family practitioner services which refer to 1 July.

[2] Staff of the Family Practitioner Committees, mass radiography units, blood transfusion centres, and Boards of Governors are included. Common Services Agency staff in Scotland are included.

[3] Figures for hospital medical and dental staff exclude locums, hospital practitioners and paragaph 94 and 107 appointments. Figures for community health staff exclude occasional sessional staff in Great Britain; Northern Ireland figures include all community sessional staff.

[4] In Northern Ireland the Central Services Agency.

Source: Department of Health and Social Security, Scottish Health Service, Common Services Agency; Welsh Office, Department of Health and Social Services, Northern Ireland

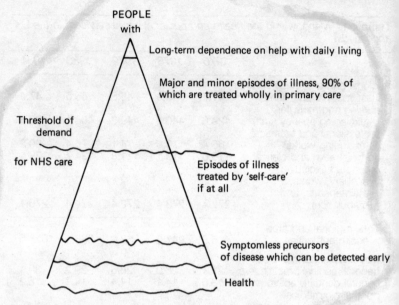

Figure 4.2 Distribution of illness and care in the UK.

Although, as can be seen, there are many more people in the groups who do not seek help than in those who do, there are several ways in which health service staff are involved in promoting the well-being of these groups. The philosophy of health promotion and illness prevention is described in Chapter 3 and only an outline of 'who does what' is given here.

Health promotion and illness prevention

It is generally accepted nowadays that no amount of action by doctors will be effective in promoting the health of individuals unless the latter accept health as an integral part of the responsibility that all of us take for our own lives and those of the fellow members of our society. Thus health promotion requires that some medical knowledge be made available to everyone rather than being handled only within the framework of doctor–patient contacts. The promotion of the public's health has two main service components. The first comprises general health education, the development of schemes of disease prevention and early detection, and monitoring of communicable diseases in man.

It is broadly termed 'community health' and is combined with a concern for health care in the speciality of community medicine. The second is the monitoring and control of the environment in which people live, environmental or public health, and is the responsibility of local government, but the health authority is required to designate a medical officer to advise and liaise with local government on this and on communicable disease control. Environmental services include water supplies, sewage and refuse disposal and air pollution.

At the level of the individual, prevention may be practised by anyone in the health service, but three groups are especially trained for this work; health visitors, a group of doctors working mainly with children outside hospital (clinical medical officers) and health education officers, whose role is to generate health education material and to stimulate health education activities by individual doctors and other health care professionals.

However, all doctors are increasingly being encouraged to use the opportunities of doctor–patient contacts to persuade people to change 'bad' habits for 'good' ones as it is generally believed that patients will be more receptive to advice at that point than when they feel well. It is not known how much of the average general practitioner's time is spent on prevention, but only about 5% of the annual expenditure of the NHS goes on identifiable preventive service (including the national health education bodies).

Self-care

This is a global term which includes activities of health promotion, treating one's own bee-stings and head colds, mutual aid for intractable problems such as chronic cystitis (such group activity is often called 'self-help'), monitoring one's own blood pressure if given medical advice so to do; indeed, any activity which might fall within the present remit of health services or might require what is sometimes thought of as 'medical' knowledge. Although people have always coped with many of their own problems and minor illnesses, there is at present a good deal of discussion about where the division should be between 'self-care,' and health services, i.e. which illnesses fall above or below the threshold of formal care. The debate concerns ethical, legal, professional and resource issues. However, it is clear that if people stopped handling many of their own and their families' illnesses, the health services would be swamped.

Primary care

The first or primary point of contact for most ill people is their general practitioner or, more accurately, the practice receptionist. The general medical practitioner is in one of four professional *primary care* or first-line services. It should be remembered that although a health authority has overall responsibility for services in an area, general practitioners remain independent contractors, i.e. they contract with health authorities to provide a service for which they are paid, but they are not accountable to the government. Instead, they are accountable to their peers and may be disciplined by them for certain acts such as unjustifiable excessive prescribing or in the case of complaints.

This category of primary care includes the following services:

General medical services (i.e. primary medical care) provided by the patient's own family doctor. The doctor is paid a 'capitation fee' for these services in respect of every person on his list, an additional sum being paid for each person over 65 years of age and a further sum for those aged 75 or more. This fee is paid on a quarterly basis, and is not related to the amount of service any particular patient may have received although, at the time of writing, there is discussion about a government proposal to pay a 'good practice allowance' to those practices which provide a wide range of desirable services. Certain services (for example, maternity care) are paid for separately as 'items of service'. A general practitioner has to have postgraduate training in obstetrics before he is permitted to undertake domiciliary midwifery. Some general practitioners, however, choose not to take on domiciliary confinements. The vast majority of people in the UK are on the list of a general practitioner of their own choice and all are free to change their doctor if they so desire. It is open to any citizen to approach a doctor on a private basis provided he is not on that doctor's NHS list.

General dental services are provided on the basis of a fee for service paid to the dentist, with certain fixed charges to the patient at the time of treatment.

General pharmaceutical services. Medicines prescribed by general practitioners under the NHS are dispensed by retail pharmacists on terms negotiated at national level by the health departments and representatives of the pharmacists. The patient is charged a fee per item on the prescription, regardless of the cost of substances prescribed, the money going to the NHS. Certain categories of patients with chronic illness, all pensioners, children and expectant mothers, have free medicine.

General ophthalmic services provide sight-testing and the supply of spectacles, for which there is a fee for service plus certain fixed charges to the recipient.

The term 'primary care team' is used to describe the general practitioner and his colleagues from other professions – the home nurse, health visitor and practice receptionist. Ideally, it contains a social worker, but very few are available to work with health services and most of those who do are based in hospital. The majority of doctors work as part of such teams and in group practices rather than singlehanded, so that the nurses, for example, can also form a group. Note that other professions, such as therapists, also visit people at home, but are called domiciliary rather than primary care staff, because they are brought in by the primary care team and are not the first point of contact of patients with the health service. Thus the focal point of all episodes of care is the primary care team.

Hospital and specialist services

Only a few general practitioners can admit patients to, and treat them in, hospital and this happens only in rural areas or in maternity units. To reach the hospital and specialist services, patients must be referred (except in an emergency) by their general practitioners. The role of the specialist service is:

(1) to advise general practitioners on special problems of diagnosis or treatment
(2) to provide services which cannot be given outside hospital
(3) to provide services which have to be coordinated to an extent that they are more efficiently organized through a central complex.

Not all doctors working in hospitals are health service employees: in teaching hospitals some are university employees with honorary contracts in the health service.

More than one-half of the NHS annual expenditure is on acute services in primary care or hospital; a further one-third goes on long-term nursing care – physical or psychiatric. There are very few nursing homes within the NHS but so far as possible, within existing hospitals, separate units or wards are adapted or designed to be less formal and more homely than acute wards can be.

Private medical and nursing care began to increase in the early 1980s because of the cutbacks in public health service spending. Private medical care decreases from south to north in Britain, being most common in the metropolitan south-east and least (less than 5% of consultant medical time) in the north of Scotland. Private acute nursing care is provided through agencies and may be bought by the hospital service (to fill gaps) or by individual patients at home. Private long-term nursing care is more usually offered in private nursing homes; these must be approved by the local health authority before a licence is granted.

Informal care

As well as choosing for themselves to stay off work or buy medicines from a chemist for minor illnesses such as colds and 'flu, people who are ill may need to be looked after at home for short or long spells. They may need simple but basic items such as meals in bed, more extensive help such as with washing and dressing after a limb injury, or total care such as is given to infants or to someone who has had a severe stroke. In most instances, family and friends assume the responsibility for helping and regard it as a normal part of family life. However, as the numbers of people requiring a great deal of long-term care have increased and the numbers of potential helpers at home have decreased (*see* Chapter 1), awareness has grown of the extent of informal care (i.e. not part of the formal health or personal social services). As with health promotion and self-care, there is now open discussion about the relative responsibility of professional services and informal supporters at home, and in awareness of the need to 'care for the carers' to prevent the breakdown of home care.

PROFESSIONS IN HEALTH CARE

The preceding outline of types of care concerns the system by which people are helped or help themselves. Within the system there are many different professions and in understanding who does what, it is useful to know a little about how they are trained and, very broadly, their respective roles. The following is in no way comprehensive, but serves as an introduction to the main professions who work with patients. The roles of doctors have been outlined above and those with whom doctors are most likely to work discussed below.

Nurses, midwives and health visitors

Nursing staff who include midwives and health visitors form the largest category of staff employed in the health service. They work not only in hospitals, but also in the community providing health care in the home to the elderly, young children and the sick.

The International Council of Nursing describes the function of nursing as follows:

> 'The unique function of the nurse is to assist the individual, sick or well, in the performance of those activities contributing to health or its recovery (or to peaceful death) that he would perform unaided if he had the necessary strength, will or knowledge; and to do this in such a way as to help him gain independence as rapidly as possible' (Henderson, 1968).

About one-half of the nursing and midwifery staff employed in the hospital service are qualified, the remainder being either nursing auxiliaries or undergoing training; in the community, virtually all nursing staff are qualified. Over recent years patient care has become more intensive and specialized, and has led to increased demands on nursing and midwifery resources.

There are several ways in which a nurse can become qualified. Colleges of Nursing and Midwifery offer 3-year courses leading to the qualification of registration with the UK Central Council in one of four specialized fields – general nursing, sick children's nursing, psychiatric nursing and mental handicap nursing. In addition, degree courses in nursing are offered at a number of universities and colleges of technology. Shorter courses of under 2 years leading to the qualification of enrolled nurse are also available, although discussions are taking place with a view to discontinuing this level of training. Postbasic courses prepare nurses to work as midwives, district nurses and health visitors and national boards examine the need for, and approve courses in, further continuing education and specialist clinical courses. At the time of writing several proposals are being discussed for a major reform of nurse education to ensure a greater emphasis on health rather than illness and a larger common core of training for different nursing specialities.

Midwives are Registered General Nurses who have successfully completed an 18-month course in midwifery. This course adequately prepares them to be independent practitioners in all aspects of pre- and postnatal care and of the normal delivery. In view of the recent trend towards hospital deliveries, most Registered Midwives are employed in that setting. However, increasing demands from clients for home deliveries are likely to result in an increase in community-based midwives.

Health visitors are particularly important in community medicine because, as well as being trained nurses with midwifery experience, they are trained health educators. Their aim is to promote health and their original responsibility was in mother and child welfare by giving advice to expectant and nursing mothers about good care of themselves and their young children, for example, feeding and diet, normal milestones of development, accident prevention and hygiene. The health visitor is concerned with the health of the family unit and, as the health of young children has improved, her (occasionally his) work has extended not only into school health, but also into primary and tertiary prevention for the chronic sick and handicapped, and increasingly the elderly. Most health visitors are now attached to general practices as part of the primary care team and may carry out secondary prevention or screening for particular problems in conjunction with the doctors in the practice.

District nurses are trained in a comparable way to health visitors. Their additional one-year course covers, in depth, subjects such as sociology, social policy and the psychology of communication. Their particular skills lie in the adaptation of professional nursing care to the individual patient in his home environment. Like health visitors, most are attached to general practices.

The trend of transferring psychiatric care, whenever possible, from hospital to the community has resulted in the development of another specialist nurse – the community psychiatric nurse. These are Registered Mental Nurses who have successfully completed a course similar in length and depth to a district nursing course.

Paramedical professions

The paramedical professions include occupational therapists, physiotherapists, remedial gymnasts, speech therapists, chiropodists, dietitians, orthoptists, radiographers, orthotists, prosthetists, dental auxiliaries and dental hygienists. Doctors are most likely to work with the 'remedial' professions – those who help patients to achieve maximum function and independence at work, at home and in society.

Treatment includes advice to patients, their relatives and other members of the rehabilitation team and may take place in hospital or elsewhere. Remedial therapists can assess and define the objectives of treatment of patients referred to them by doctors, although the latter remain in clinical charge. Most have 3-years' training leading to state registration and there is an increasing number of degree courses at universities and colleges of technology. Each remedial profession offers particular skills.

Occupational therapists help people to learn, or relearn, the skills of daily living used in personal care, work or family and social roles. The philosophy of occupational therapy is based on problem solving. They assess and treat patients of all age groups whose function is impaired physically, psychologically or socially. A wide range of techniques is used depending on the particular problem and the patient's own environment. For example, the techniques may be physical, such as individually designed simple aids, or psychological, such as motivating the patient to take decisions about shopping. The NHS remains the major employing authority for occupational therapists, although an increasing number of therapists are now being employed within Departments of Social Work. A small number work with voluntary agencies, in special schools and other organizations, as well as in schools of occupational therapy.

Physiotherapists help people to gain or regain physical independence after illness or injury. They use specific exercise techniques designed to promote and develop particular activities and functions, for example, rehabilitation following stroke or the finely skilled movements following hand surgery. They also use a number of techniques such as mobilization, electrical and heat treatment and massage in the treatment of local joint disorders, pain and associated problems. Physiotherapy is used preventively most commonly in the treatment of surgical patients to prevent respiratory and circulatory complications and in ante- and postnatal care. They are also involved in teaching lifting and handling skills in the prevention of back injury and in the prevention of deformities and maintenance of activities in the severely handicapped child and adult.

Increasing numbers of physiotherapists work outside the hospital, usually in the patients' homes where their task is to assess patients' physical capabilities and, in cooperation with the family and primary care team, set up relevant exercise programmes which can be carried out and monitored in the home in the absence of the therapist.

Speech therapists are experts in communication problems arising from disease, injury, deafness or emotional difficulties and their skills are relevant to all types of dysfunction of communication whether it be in understanding or in expression, oral or written. They have to understand the structure of language as well as cerebral and neurological pathways.

The majority of speech therapists work with children and are employed by the health service, although some work in schools. A large part of the work is with preschool children, including those who for any reason have not started to speak at an appropriate age. However, increasing numbers work with adults and in hospital, mainly treating patients with neurological disorders, voice disorders or with difficulties of articulation following ENT surgery.

Dietitians apply the science of nutrition to the needs of both healthy and ill people. Most of them work in hospitals where their main task is the provision of diets modified in consistency or in nutrient content. Patients awaiting surgery or who have undergone surgery may require a modified diet in addition to those patients suffering from liver, renal or coeliac disease, diabetes, inborn errors of metabolism (such as phenylketonuria) or obesity.

Recently, dietitians have become involved in supervising the nutritional content of patient and staff meals and in organizing and implementing district food policies.

Dietitians also work in the community where their main role is the prevention of nutritionally related disorders in all age groups. Some are involved in clinics in health centres, but they also provide advice and nutritional information for health visitors, home economists, school meals' organizers, general practitioners, social workers and health education officers.

Most dietitians are employed by the health service, but some are employed as teachers at various levels of education and some health education officers are dietetically qualified. Some dietitians work in the food industry.

Social workers

Training is usually either 2 or 4 years and may take non-graduate, undergraduate or postgraduate forms at either colleges of technology or universities and covers all the responsibilities outlined in the section on Social work, (*see* p. 102).

Social workers are employed by local Social Service Departments in England and Wales, by Regional Authority Departments of Social Work in Scotland and by Health and Social Services Boards in Northern Ireland. A small proportion work in voluntary agencies, e.g. Dr Barnardo's. Teams of caseworkers deal with a vast range of problems arising from homelessness, familial deprivation, poverty, criminality, illness, handicap and ageing. They also liaise with other community sources of help such as doctors, housing officers, DHSS, Courts, the police and the children's hearings system. Residential social workers practise in a more specialized way with particular groups, e.g. the elderly, the disturbed and the handicapped. Other specialities include youth and community work, and community education.

The group of social workers with whom doctors work most closely are those based in hospitals, and/or linked to health centres and group practices. There is a tendency among health service staff to regard social workers mainly as sources of 'welfare' provision such as home helps or housing adaptations, but social workers define their task rather differently:

'Social work is a professional service based on the understanding of the psychosocial implications of illness and handicap. All patients who face the problems of physical helplessness, deformity and mutilation, incurable progressive illness and death, experience anxiety, fear, loss and grief. They have a responsibility to know and understand the medical situation and the implications of this for the patient and his family, the problems they present for them and the potential stresses they bring. Medical social work can be preventive in help given with foresight of the probable social consequences for the patient and his family, including mobilizing practical resources and services on his behalf. Unless medical social workers are an essential part of the health service they cannot fulfil their role of helping sick people and their families to adjust to illness and its treatment, nor counter the overwhelming sense for many patients and their families of isolation, depression, loss and bereavement.' (HMSO, 1974).

The following are examples of common areas of joint medical and social work involvement.

Mothers and young children	Family planning: single parents; teenage mothers; battered babies; handicapped; families under stress; adoption

Children – school age	Early recognition of handicap; solvent abuse and problems of addiction; young offenders
– school leavers	Employment of handicapped and maladjusted; adaptation to unemployment
Adults	Chronic debilitating illness; severe loss of physical function; disfigurement–deformity; personality disorder
Elderly	Suitable housing; loneliness; restricted mobility; community support; placement in long-term care.

Clinical psychologists

Clinical psychologists work with patients of all ages who have psychological or behavioural difficulties, which may arise as a result of physical illness or injury as well as from non-organic factors, or who are mentally handicapped. They have a degree in general psychology followed by a postgraduate course in clinical applications of psychology. They use these techniques both in assessing and treating patients and also, with other health care professions, in devising, applying and evaluating programmes of care for people with long-term problems such as psychotic or demented patients. They work in a variety of speciality settings such as psychiatry, mental handicap, child health, community services, general medicine, neurology, geriatrics and rehabilitation.

LOCAL AUTHORITY SERVICES

Housing Acts

These require all local authorities to inspect the houses in their areas to prevent overcrowding and to ensure their maintenance in good repair. Environmental health officers carry out this, following 2 years special training which also enables them to supervise new building.

Local authorities may condemn houses as unfit for human

habitation, and may clear or redevelop whole slum areas (Town Planning Department). They are responsible for rehousing these families and for assisting homeless people.

These Acts also authorize the building of 'council' houses to be rented by the public. A housing department organizes the building and renting of these dwellings, operating a waiting-list with a points system for advancement based on social and medical factors contributing to need for rehousing.

The Clean Air Act

The emission of dark smoke from any chimney is an offence under the Clean Air Act which requires all local authorities to enforce the prohibition, through the environmental health officers. In addition, local authorities may declare smoke control areas (colloquially known as 'smokeless zones') in which it is forbidden to emit any smoke from chimneys – domestic, industrial or locomotive. The local authority may pay up to 70% of the cost of approved adaptation of domestic appliances for the burning of smokeless fuel.

The Education Acts

These require local education authorities to provide a school health service to examine the children at intervals and to ensure that treatment is available for any defect found. Clinics for the treatment of minor ailments, ENT, eye and orthopaedic abnormalities are provided. Health visitors act as school nurses for the examinations and, for the treatments, may be assisted by clinic nurses.

The Act permits education authorities to provide *Child Guidance Clinics* for handicapped, backward and difficult children, to be able to advise parents and teachers about their education and to provide the special educational treatment that may be needed. Child and adolescent psychiatrists from the NHS cooperate with educational psychologists in these clinics.

Special education

Under the Education Acts, a child with any form of learning difficulty (except a difference of language between home and school) is defined as having special educational needs. Local education authorities must find and assess all such children and, bearing in mind the views of the parents, arrange an appropriate educational placement. This may be in an ordinary school (with or without special facilities), a special school, or a hospital. It is the accepted principle that no child should be in a special school if his other needs can be met in an ordinary school. However, special schools provide education of the type and at the pace suited to the needs of each handicapped child. For certain handicaps, for example, blindness, the child may have to go to a residential special school where the facilities are shared by several education authorities.

Social Services Acts

Departments of social services or social work within local authorities have the following responsibilities.

Care of children

Local authorities must provide for children who are deprived of a normal home life, (Powers under the Children and Young Persons Acts 1963 and 1969 and Child Care Act, 1980) including:

(1) coordination of services for unmarried mothers and one-parent families
(2) registration of adoption societies and the supervision of children awaiting adoption
(3) supervision of child minders and private foster parents, private day and residential nurseries
(4) residential and day nurseries for children requiring such accommodation on social or health grounds
(5) care proceedings brought by a local authority if it believes that a child is in need of improved care.

Statutory grounds for care are:

(1) the child is beyond the control of the parents
(2) through lack of parental care, the child is falling into bad associations or is exposed to moral danger, suffering or ill-health
(3) a specified criminal offence has been committed against him or her and, if female, that she may be at risk of an incestuous offence
(4) failure to attend school regularly

(5) commission of an offence, including referral from a court (previously the probation procedure).

Anyone may refer or report a child's circumstances for investigation. The juvenile court (in Scotland, the children's panel), if it considers it desirable, may make a supervision requirement to place the child under supervision or care, either at home, in a day or residential centre or in hospital.

Care and after-care (other than medical care)

Under this heading are:

(1) non-medical services for those who are or have been suffering from illness, e.g. provision of home helps, occupational therapists
(2) welfare of the chronically sick and the disabled (formerly the National Assistance Act, 1948). *The Chronically Sick and Disabled Persons Act, 1970* extended this remit to include the setting up of a regular publication of information about existing services, and the provision of access for the disabled to all public buildings
(3) residential care for the relatively healthy elderly who need no more medical or nursing care than would be provided in their own homes (formerly National Assistance Act, Part III and known as 'Part III Accommodation').

VOLUNTARY AGENCIES

There are two basic categories of voluntary agencies – self-help groups and agencies who help other people. Voluntary organizations are financed and run independently, but many cooperate with, and indeed receive grants from, local government and health authorities.

Self-help groups consist of affected people, and their relatives and friends, who help and support each other, usually without the help of professionals such as doctors or social workers. The best known example is Alcoholics Anonymous; others are 'U and I' clubs (for cystitis sufferers) or the Ileostomy Association.

The second type of voluntary agency sets out to help others rather than its own members. Two well known examples are The Samaritans and the WRVS (Women's Royal Voluntary Service) which provides among other things 'meals-on-wheels'.

There are very many voluntary agencies, both local and national, of which the following are a few prominent examples.

The Old People's Welfare Council provides old people's homes, flats and clubs, as well as arranging other forms of recreation and a 'meals-on-wheels' service. In many areas it has changed its name to *Age Concern*. A home visiting service to bring companionship to the housebound, and a night-sitter service for the terminal stages of prolonged illness are just two of the many services designed to help infirm people to remain in their own homes. Recently, it has developed a growing interest in supporting the families who look after elderly people at home.

The Citizen's Advice Bureau exists to help solve everyday difficulties and to show how specialist help can be obtained for the more complex ones. It is also intended as a guide to the public through the ever-increasing tangle of local and central government administration and legislation.

Alcoholics Anonymous is an association of alcoholics, formed to try to help each other to control their drinking. Moral support without any 'holier-than-thou' aspect has had some effect. The services of the association are for members only, but if an alcoholic wishes to join, he simply goes to a meeting.

The Samaritans give help to anyone who feels he is being overwhelmed by his difficulties, no matter what they are. One of the main purposes is to help people who are near to suicide, and so they must be available at any time.

Mind (National Association for Mental Health) campaigns for the needs and rights of mentally ill and mentally handicapped people. It also provides a social work advisory service for patients and their families as well as running educational and research programmes.

SERVICES FOR CHILDREN AND OLD PEOPLE

Useful examples of the interplay and overlap of the services so far described can be obtained by discussing their relevance to particular groups of patients.

Children and handicap

The pattern of serious disease in children has changed over the past 40 years from mainly acute illness usually requiring one prolonged episode of hospital care to mainly chronic illness and handicap with several hospital admissions and the involvement of multidisciplinary teams. These teams are necessary to ensure satisfactory long-term care and, in addition to various medical and nursing specialities, will include a physiotherapist, occupational therapist, psychologist, teacher and social worker.

Measurements of children's health have traditionally been mortality rates, but morbidity rates have now become more relevant (*see* Information Services, p. 38). The still-birth rate and the perinatal mortality rate give an indication of the effectiveness of the obstetric services of an area. The infant mortality rate is related to the general standard of living in an area or country. All these rates have shown a considerable decrease over the past 30 years, but have levelled out at rates above those for Scandinavian countries. Even within the UK there is variation, for example according to urban/rural residence and social class. Thus, although improvement has occurred, there are still sections of the population which would benefit from increased health service provision, usually in association with improvement in housing and other environmental factors.

The general practitioner, in association with the health visitor, provides continuing care and supervision for all children. In most areas developmental screening programmes are available from birth, provided partly by general practitioners and partly by doctors with a special interest in child health.

Again, it should be noted that not all parents avail themselves of this service and, since in general those most in need are included in the defaulters and since it is important to detect any handicapping condition as early as possible, follow-up of the non-attenders is necessary. Assessment centres exist to investigate in greater detail those children suspected of being handicapped. The school health service is responsible for identifying all school-age children whose education may suffer because of a physical or mental condition, and for ensuring that any disability is alleviated whenever possible. In some instances this is best achieved by providing special educational facilities, especially in cases of mental handicap.

An outline of the services relevant to Child Health is given in Fig. 4.3.

Students should therefore be aware of the changing pattern of disease in children and of the importance of multidisciplinary teams in caring for the chronically ill and handicapped. They should also be

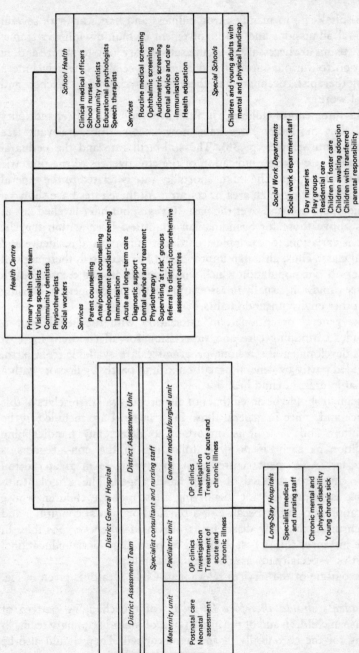

Figure 4.3 Child health and paediatric services.

School Health

Clinical medical officers
School nurses
Community dentists
Educational psychologists
Speech therapists

Services

Routine medical screening
Ophthalmic screening
Audiometric screening
Dental advice and care
Immunisation
Health education

Special Schools

Children and young adults with mental and physical handicap

Social Work Departments

Social work department staff

Day nurseries
Play groups
Residential care
Children in foster care
Children awaiting adoption
Children with transferred parental responsibility

Health Centre

Primary health care team
Visiting specialists
Community dentists
Physiotherapists
Social workers

Services

Parent counselling
Ante/postnatal counselling
Development paediatric screening
Immunisation
Acute and long-term care
Dental advice and treatment
Diagnostic support
Physiotherapy
Supervising 'at risk' groups
Referral to district/comprehensive assessment centres

District General Hospital

District Assessment Team

District Assessment Unit

Specialist consultant and nursing staff

Maternity unit

Postnatal care
Neonatal assessment

Paediatric unit

OP clinics
Investigation
Treatment of acute and chronic illness

General medical/surgical unit

OP clinics
Investigation
Treatment of acute and chronic illness

Long-Stay Hospitals

Specialist medical and nursing staff

Chronic mental and physical disability
Young chronic sick

aware of the differential uptake of child health service and the effects of this.

They should know:

(1) the measures of health and ill-health in children
(2) the organization of health services available for all children including development screening programmes and school health service
(3) the categories of handicap and the services available for handicapped children including the non-health agencies and personnel involved.

Older people

One of the biggest issues facing society today is how to adapt to the increasing proportion of retired and elderly people both before and when they become in need of medical care. Fifteen per cent of the population is aged 65 or more and nearly one-half of these are aged over 75. In the next 25 years, it is estimated that although the 65–74 age group will decrease, the 85+ age group will increase by about 50%.

The likely impact of this change in population both on older people themselves and on the services which might help them can be examined by reference to the questions in Chapter 2, namely:

(1) what are we trying to achieve?
(2) what is happening now?
(3) what is the best way to reach our objectives?

What are we trying to achieve?

Ideals for the care of elderly people were proposed by the Royal College of Physicians of Edinburgh in 1963 and later adopted by the World Health Organization. They are:

(1) to sustain them in independence, comfort and contentment in their own homes and, when independence begins to wane, to support them by all necessary means for as long as possible
(2) to offer alternative residential accommodation to those who, by reasons of age, infirmity, lack of a proper home, or other circumstances, are in need of care and attention
(3) to provide, promptly, hospital accommodation for those who, by

reason of physical or mental ill health, are in need of a full medical assessment, therapy, rehabilitation, or long-term skilled medical and/or nursing care.

These criteria are widely used by health authorities and professions in planning services with the addition of a fourth ideal, namely, 'to help everyone to withdraw from life with as much dignity and comfort as possible'. Like most ideals, they describe the direction in which services should go, but not the precise objectives for each area. Before they can be specified, for areas which differ, we need to know some of the answers to the second question so that the precise objectives are realistic.

What is happening now?

Older people are high users of all services. First, the risk of acute illness increases with age (after the first year of life); second, biological ageing causes slower recovery from acute illness; and third, older people tend to have multiple disease and functional problems and also to live alone.

Thus those over the age of 74, who are about 6% of the population, account for 14% of all hospital admissions, but about half of the beds used (acute and long-term combined). Several points arise from this: first, that older people should be expected to take a few days longer than the average to recover from an acute illness, whether at home or in an acute ward. Second, that the term 'services for the elderly' refers to those services which are geared to the particular combination of problems experienced in later life and especially after the age of 75. Third, that even after the age of 75, the majority of people regard themselves as healthy and it is only a small proportion (less than 10%) who have a need for long-term care.

Another factor is that the changing balance of population means that there are fewer young people to provide short-term or small items of informal support. More married women than formerly have jobs outside the home, and there is selective survival to old age of women who were not exposed to childbirth and, of course, who are childless. It is not true to say that 'families don't care', but it is true that their availability is less. It may also be true that older people now expect to be independent and do not take family support for granted: 'I don't want to be a burden' is a common statement. For all these reasons the formal services, which follow a pattern similar to that shown for children in Fig. 4.3 (*see* p. 106), now provide a wider range of types of paramedical help than in the past. For example, home nurses and domiciliary therapists spend most of their time with old people.

Social work departments provide care in residential homes, the home help service, wardens for sheltered housing (the housing itself is provided and allocated by district housing departments), occupational therapists to assess the need for aids and adaptations in the home; the aids, including telephones and alarm systems are also provided by these departments. They are responsible for knowing about all the handicapped elderly in their region so that they can, for example, provide emergency heating during a power cut, and for ensuring that the elderly are informed about services available to help them.

Confusion may arise between health and local authority services about who is to provide certain physical aids and about which facility – sheltered housing, residential home or hospital – is most suitable for a particular elderly person. Hence a system of multi-professional assessment of patients is essential to ensure that they are most aptly cared for and that gaps and overlaps between services are eliminated.

The needs that arise with ageing differ from those in younger people because of the interaction of the several clinical entities and because there is a greater emphasis on the patient's capacity to function within his particular environment. Older people tend to stay in their original housing and they more often live alone. Thus the balance can be easily disrupted by minor illness, so that someone who is coping well on his or her own may become very dependent on help from outside simply because of influenza or an infected toe-nail. In Fig. 4.4 the most common problems and services are listed alongside the trend of increasing dependence. The most common clinical problems are arthritis (of all types) and depression or anxiety, with dementia next in frequency. These give rise to successive types of need for help with functioning: an easier physical environment, help with mobility, with housework and with personal care such as washing and dressing. Also, elderly people themselves want to have one or two close friends or visitors with whom they can form a relationship.

The factors in an old person which cause greatest stress on families and friends who are helping at home are night confusion (and hence sleep disturbance for the household), faecal incontinence, being bed-

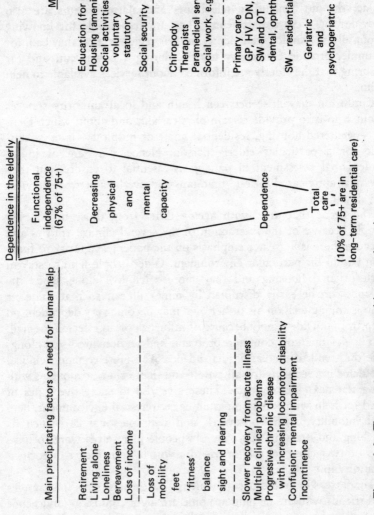

Figure 4.4 The most common problems and services.

fast, or restrictions on the helpers' social life. These factors thus result in an increased likelihood of seeking help from services.

What is the best way to achieve our objectives?

As indicated earlier, the precise targets for numbers of staff or institutional places will vary between areas and will depend in part on the priority put locally on care of the elderly compared with other groups (the 'how much can we afford?' question). There are also differences in policy. In England and Wales, there is much greater emphasis on local government residential care than in Scotland. As a result, the target rate of provision of geriatric hospital beds is much lower in England and Wales. However, universal aspects in which there is need for improvement and which would permit best use of each area's resources are:

(1) research into causes of dementia, arthritis, etc. (so that prevention becomes possible) and into bioengineering methods of aiding disabled people
(2) a new housing policy so that frail people can move about in any house
(3) support for families and communities so that they can share responsibilities and seek help from services before crisis occurs
(4) seeking an agreed policy for control of institutions and admissions to places or beds so that inappropriate placement is avoided
(5) education of staff in new ways of delivering acute care and redistribution of beds
(6) increasing awareness of all ages in society to the nature and effects of Western attitudes to old age.

Students should know:
(1) the demographic reasons for the increase in the proportion of elderly people in the population
(2) the social changes in the past few decades which have increased the demand for care of the elderly by health and social services
(3) the effects of biological, psychological and social ageing on the illness process in old people
(4) the environmental hazards for old people living at home
(5) the medical conditions common in the elderly, including those likely to be unrecognized by the elderly person, and the fact that the presentation of illness is often unusual

(6) the particular groups of elderly people at high risk of needing care and advice at home and of institutionalization
(7) the effects on the family of caring for an increasingly dependent elderly person
(8) the services, health and other, which should be available to prevent dependence and to maintain an elderly person in his own home
(9) the philosophy of and services for care of the dying.

RESOURCES, CHOICES AND DECISION-MAKING

The government's policy for the balance and direction of the health service was described on p. 83. How government policy is translated into the distribution of services in a village or area is a concern for everyone in the health service, as well as those who may use it. This part of the Study Guide contains an outline of who is involved in deciding who should have how much of what. This is by no means a simple and clear-cut process; many decisions are not obvious and few are agreed by all. It is very important for their future work that students understand why this is so and, therefore, it is worth commenting first on the nature of choices before outlining the network of decision-making.

The nature of choice

At the time the health service was created, the ideal was to provide the best possible medical care for everyone but, in reality, resources have been, are and always will be scarce. Choices have to be made of what to do and therefore of what not to do. The public, patients, professionals and planners all have an interest in seeing that the resources that do exist are used to the best effect. People inevitably disagree on whether the choices which are made reflect the 'proper' value of what is best. With private medicine each consumer chooses the best use of his own resources according to his values at that time. In a national system the emphasis changes; the consumer no longer buys just what he wants and the responsibility for weighing up the alternative uses of his and everyone else's money lies with the government and its representatives or nominees at local level. Because the choices of which services to provide and which not to provide are taken on his behalf, however indirectly, the consumer has a right to know the bases on which they are made. It may be possible to reach a consensus of values which are shared by both the health services and the consumers, but nonetheless the relative values being applied by the health services should be made explicit to the people who are paying for them.

How can we determine values – how can we agree on how much money should be spent on health services? It is certainly true that less is available than could be used, but it would also be true that spending more would make very little difference to the vast majority of *deaths* which, despite more money, would still occur. Of course, a few deaths might be avoided or delayed, but virtually all the additional expenditure would have to be set against the few additional lives saved; and implicitly by spending the money that would become the value of those lives.

If, on the other hand, the aim were to reduce *illness*, not just death, would we fare better? Unfortunately, this too is unlikely for, as we know, many of our diseases and deaths are partly of our own making (smoking, obesity, addiction, pollution) with the damage already done. To avoid this by prevention would mean action with the young, with the costs now and the benefits delayed for two or more decades. Even then, if *prevention* is the aim, it is questionable whether this ought to be an expansion of the health service, since the troubles lie in the environment and in our habits. All that could be done now is to increase the care, rather than the cure, for those who are already disabled.

Nonetheless, there are these three purposes for which more resources (were the public to agree they should be made available) could be used by the health services and if there is not money for all three, which should carry the priority and what should the balance be amongst them? And, more difficult, who should decide that priority?

The argument is frequently made that such choices are virtually impossible or at the very least are totally unreasonable. However, even in life-threatening conditions resources are not pumped in indefinitely; there comes a point when it is obvious that resources are being taken away from another activity so that the benefit of lives saved in the one is less than the number of lives lost in the other. Different trade-offs can be identified at different margins and at different levels, first within life-threatening conditions and second between life-threatening conditions and those providing care and comfort. Here, the direction of the trade-offs may not always be that which superficial consideration might suggest. Death under some circumstances may well carry less priority when set against years of living in suffering; it is as already indicated, a matter of personal and social values.

Today the main difficulties centre on achieving a proper distribution of resources between the various services – between the acute and non-acute hospital services, between the hospital and community services, and between care and prevention. At present the hospitals offer acute care and save lives; but the problem is that many of these patients then require continuing care which, frankly, at the present moment is inadequate. Given these demands what remains for prevention and for the future?

There is much said about the need to expand the community services such as medical, nursing, financial, advisory and employment services; domestic help, meals on wheels, physiotherapy, occupational therapy, social work, chiropody, the simple aids (e.g. walking machines, bed pans and laundry) that can be made available in the patients' homes. Many of these services are often taken for granted in hospital, but they absorb a large amount of health service and local authority resources. There is no question about the need for hospital care, the questions are the amount, its costs, its form and its organization. There have been tremendous developments over the last 20 years and paradoxically while providing a whole series of achievements in terms of technical care, they have created an additional and costly burden for the health service. On the other hand, a consideration of need (caused by an increasing disabled and ageing population) may not please the medical profession because the new services that should be developed may not match the current impression of what scientific and technical medical care of the future should be. The need now is to face up to these choices and find a means of sharing the responsibility for the care of the chronic sick and the elderly, and ways of detecting treatable disease as early as possible, so that the best possible use is made of resources.

Arguments about the need for further services or that the present ones could be more effective are all very well, but how are the resources used now? The cost of the NHS increases annually with the largest amount being spent on hospitals, and in hospitals nearly two-thirds going on salaries. The rising costs have come about for a number of reasons: these include shorter working weeks, higher salaries, increased expectations of patients and improved treatment. The hoped for reduction in costs from creating a healthy nation has simply not materialized.

The answer is not just more money – the total at present is not unreasonable. It is always possible to spend more, but first we have to be sure that what is available now is being spent properly – the real problem is that we do not know how it is being spent. This arose because when the health service started there was a genuine fear that care would be unduly restricted by cost; this was safe-guarded by preserving what was called clinical freedom, i.e. the right for doctors to determine the care appropriate for patients unfettered by cost considerations. To preserve this freedom, the provision of budgets for clinical services was deemed inappropriate and, indeed, the present accounting system makes it very difficult to relate the costs of the resources used to the care given to individual patients or even groups of patients. Clinical budgets are now being introduced as part of a management reorganization (*see* p. 116), but there is no plan to include routinely information about clinical outcomes. Somehow, we have to find out more about what is being achieved in terms of improved health for the resources that are being used. In the meantime, judgements are made by government in the light of competing claims for exchequer funds, and here we come back to the essential concepts of choice and values. We spend more now than 10 years ago, much more than 20 years ago, but maybe less than in 10 years time. What is allocated to the health service is relative to the values of society at that time.

In addition, every decision, at every level of living and working, is a choice, even a refusal to choose is a passive choice. People do not always realize this. The financial situation in the NHS can be likened to an enormous raft. After a certain number of people are aboard no one else can board without pushing someone else off the other side. If it is a very big raft those climbing on (or being pushed on) may not see the people falling off the other side, may not realize anyone is falling off and, indeed, may not think anyone has to fall off. Even if the raft is made a little bigger, the problem very quickly returns. There are three aspects of this analogy that are worth noting. First, there is the size of the raft and that has very little to do with the health service, that is a problem for the government and the public. Second, there is the matter of who should board the raft, and that is a problem of the values already referred to; this is only in part a responsibility of the health service, but because these issues have not so far been made sufficiently explicit they have, perhaps wrongly, been left entirely to the health service to try to decide. Third, there is how many people can be packed onto the raft, and that is a problem of organization and planning which falls squarely on the shoulders of the health service and, therefore, represents the main components of the community medicine course. Indeed, this matter of who should decide and how to decide is the nub of health service decision-making and it is important that everyone understands where responsibility lies for various kinds of decisions.

The organization and operation of the NHS

Administrative structure

The precise structure through which the NHS is managed, from central government policy to day-to-day administration at working level, changes from time to time and varies among the component counties of the UK. In Fig. 4.5 the main elements are summarized and compared. Differences are due to a mixture of size, history and ease of communication. For example, the regional level in England is broadly equivalent to the national level in the other three countries. In the latter, there are national 'common services' organizations to provide technical support to area health agencies which it would be uneconomic to organize separately within each area, but which are provided in England at regional level. Because general practitioners are independent contractors (*see* p. 92), the administration of the primary health care services is slightly different from the rest of the NHS. In England and Wales there are autonomous Family Practitioner Committees, covering one or more districts, which are responsible for administering practitioners' contracts and for planning the four primary care services. In Scotland and Northern Ireland the administration of primary health care is undertaken by the NHS. In practice, the planning of primary health care is not well integrated with that of other services although, at the time of writing, closer coordination is being pursued by the government.

Management and staff

In 1983, an NHS management inquiry identified a lack of leadership in the NHS and recommended the introduction of general managers at all administrative levels. Some of the appointees – although not as

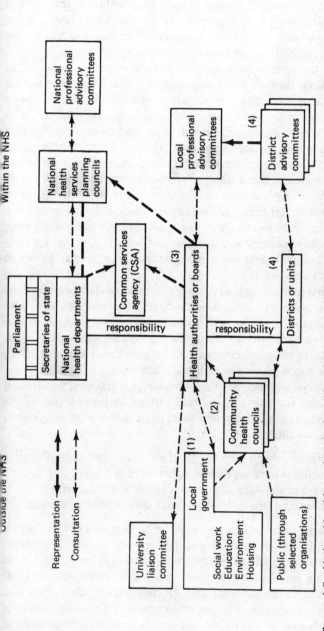

Figure 4.5 National health services in the UK: main features. (1) In Northern Ireland, personal social services (i.e. social work) are run by the same department as is health (2) In Northern Ireland, community representation is through district committees who also have a responsibility for personal social services. (3) In England, there are 14 regions which contain 195 districts. In Scotland and Wales, there are 15 and 9 areas, respectively, and in Northern Ireland there are 4 health and social service boards. (4) Only in England.

many as the government wished – were from industry, others from existing health services management. At the time of writing it is too soon to know what impact this management change has had on the direction of the NHS or on staff.

Arguably the level of most concern to future doctors is the one in whose decisions they are likely to participate, which is unit or district management. Units may encompass a geographical area or a functional speciality, such as child health. Usually, there is a community physician, nurse, administrator and (sometimes) finance officer in each unit management team. The role of doctors in giving advice (the advisory structure) or in the management structure is unlikely to increase, but a number of doctors are becoming budget-holders under a new system of management budgeting. A management or, in the case of wards and clinical departments, a clinical budget is a plan of expenditure to meet workload, usually over the coming year. As this is a new concept for doctors, and others, it is not yet fully developed, but will certainly involve doctors to a greater extent in relating costs to patients.

There exists in the health service a complex set of staff organizations (one million people in the UK with diverse professional, craft and trade backgrounds). These staff organizations have evolved over a long time – organizations such as the BMA, the Nursing Councils, Associations of Physiotherapists, Radiographers, Dentists (BDA), Pharmacists and a whole range of trade unions.

These associations look after staff welfare, i.e. training, registration and standards. They have a vital role and are an integral part of the structure. In spite of their diversity these organizations can be grouped into three main categories:

(1) administrators (who because of their immediate administrative responsibilities have no formal rights to be consulted as a group)
(2) health care professions (the core of the advisory structure)
(3) support services (the core of the joint consultative structure).

The declared management policy of the NHS since 1974 has been a partnership involving staff in the preliminary stages of decision making. Therefore, in framing policy, an authority or board has to accommodate seven major advisory groups, a community or local health council in each district and 17 individual trade unions and consultative committees. The intention was to let the advice of the medical profession be seen alongside that from other groups and the implementation has had its difficulties; for example, the advisory groups are distinct, so that nurses, doctors, dentists and paramedicals all give their advice separately. The paradox of this is that they work together as teams and then split up to give advice. The result is not totally satisfactory. Certainly, there is greater involvement, but there is no mechanism for dealing with conflicting advice except to initiate yet another round of separate consultations. In the end, those whose advice is rejected feel aggrieved. Often the outcome is a manipulated compromise (so everyone feels aggrieved). This is perhaps inevitable because now the structure makes differences over values and attitudes explicit. Conflict has always been there, only now it is not suppressed. What people sometimes forget is that it can never be different. Competition must breed conflict. But what *can* change is what staff compete for. Is it the welfare of patients or of themselves? Whose benefit is reflected in the advice on priorities?

It is not the purpose of community medicine to question the values which shape the choices made by society and the people working in the health service. The responsibility of community medicine is to detail the implications and alternatives so that the issues involved and the choices made are clearly understood by all.

Management and the public

As well as membership of health authorities, *community (local) health councils* exist in an attempt to ensure that local people have a chance to comment on their health services.

The members are appointed from voluntary organizations, local authorities, trade union movements and other bodies which may represent the community's interests in the health service. These councils have the right:

(1) to consider questions relating to the health services in their area, whether or not so asked by the authority, and to advise the authority about them, including new developments and proposed closures
(2) to visit establishments administered by the authority (this does not include practitioners' surgeries, but does include health centres)
(3) to ask for and receive information from the authority.

As with the rest of the advisory structure, health councils are not involved in the actual decisions, but must be consulted in the preliminaries; the aim is to ensure consumer participation but it is an uneasy relationship with yet another source of advice to be set against or alongside that of the staff. However, after a difficult start when they were created in 1974, most health councils are now recognized by local people as their voice to their local health services.

The public also has an arbiter, in an independent *Health Service Commissioner* or Ombudsman. His function, as prescribed by the 1900 Act, is to investigate complaints from members of the public that they have suffered injustice or hardship as a result of the services provided and against which no other redress is available. There are certain issues, however, which he may not investigate, including impending civil action, matters of clinical judgements and any action taken by the independent general medical, dental, ophthalmic or pharmaceutical practitioner, for whom there are separate complaints tribunals.

SOCIAL SECURITY

Social security is a term used to describe the many services and benefits, that are available to all citizens. National Insurance, which involves contribution for old age pensions, the health service and various benefits payable on unemployment, maternity, incapacity for work due to ill health and to industrial injury, is administered for the whole of the UK by the Department of Health and Social Security.

An up-to-date detailed guide to the benefits available is contained in *The Family Welfare Association's 'Guide to the Social Services'*. The rates of benefit vary from time to time and if details of these are required reference should be made to the current pamphlets published by the Department of Health and Social Security.

The Department of Health and Social Security has local officers, one of whom is always available, who will arrange accommodation and provide help in the form of cash, or more often kind, in an emergency. Out of normal working hours they can be contacted through the police.

The following list gives a brief indication of the kinds of cash benefits which patients may be receiving.

Sickness benefit. A flat rate of benefit paid to an insured person who is certified unfit for work by his doctor.

Invalidity pension replaces sickness benefit after long continuous entitlement. There can also be a supplementary *invalidity allowance* for people with long-term incapacity.

Maternity benefits. There are two types and an expectant mother may receive both, a *grant* to help with the expense and which is available to all, and an *allowance* if she gives up work because of pregnancy.

Death grant. A lump sum to assist with funeral expenses of an insured person.

Attendance allowance, payable to a person who requires a considerable degree of care for at least 6 months. An *invalid care allowance* is payable, in addition, to certain carers of severely disabled people.

Mobility allowance, payable to a person who is unable to walk because of physical disablement.

Industrial injuries and diseases. Industrial injury benefit, larger in amount than sickness benefit, is paid for absence from work because of an accident at work or a prescribed industrial disease (*see* Chapter 2). Disablement benefit, when appropriate, is paid when injury benefit ceases and may be supplemented by special hardship allowance or constant attendance allowance.

Exemption from prescription charges. Those eligible include everyone under 16 and over retirement age; during pregnancy; low income groups; war pensioners; and people with certain medical conditions requiring prolonged medication.

INTERNATIONAL HEALTH CARE SYSTEMS

Different countries have evolved their own systems of health care which reflect not only the medical problems prevailing in that country but also the social and economic conditions. Since the 1950s, there has been a tendency for less industrialized countries to invest in 'western' medical technology in the belief that this would bring rapid improvement in their state of health. (There are notable exceptions such as China.) It is now widely recognized that such technology is inappropriate for their major health problems, such as communicable disease and malnutrition and many countries are trying to reverse the trend. Efforts are directed at various levels in different countries: in some (e.g. Cuba and Tanzania) they are associated with changes in national ideologies, in others, rural health care is being developed as a form of care separate from that in urban areas (e.g. Iran, Venezuela), while a third group (e.g. India) consists of small, local projects in

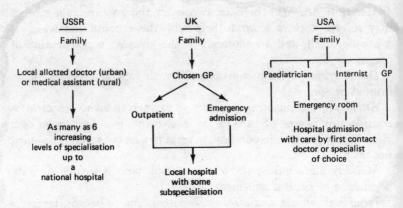

Figure 4.6 Levels of care in selected countries.

which health is only one component of a programme of community development.

Interestingly, in few are any of these basic means of providing health care actually new concepts, it is just that the attitudes and values now pertaining in that country make them acceptable, and thereby workable. It is against this background that the World Health Organization is now promoting *Health for All by the Year 2000* (pp. 78 and 153).

It is also of interest to compare and contrast the systems developed by three countries, namely, the USSR, the UK and the USA (Fig. 4.6). The main points of comparison are:

(1) emphasis on self-care and prevention
(2) degree of central control and planning
(3) the amount of continuity of care
(4) the use of medical assistants, nurses and doctors
(5) the emphasis on community versus hospital
(6) the question of private versus state medicine.

Freedom of access to different types of specialists is an issue which recurs throughout. The USA is used to represent individualism, the USSR to represent collectivism, the UK as mid-way between the two extremes and Table 4.2 summarizes some of the major differences between the three countries.

Table 4.2 *Comparison of some factors*

	USSR	UK	USA
Central control	+++	++	+(Medicare)
Continuity of care	– – –	over time	over episode
Prevention	+++	+	++(private only)
Professional freedom	– – –	+	+++
Hospital beds per 10 000 population			
all	120	80	60
psychiatric	12	40	12
OP:IP ratio	42:1	3:1	1.5:1
Manpower per 10 000 population (approx)			
doctors	30	15	17
nurses	50	80	64
medical assistants	21	0	<1
doctors (%) who are			
women	70	30	10
in general practice	25	50	20
non clinical	25	5	25
Medical graduates p.a.	12	4	4
Health indicators:			
life expectancy at birth	69	73	73
infant mortality	27	11	12
population 75+ (%)	3	6	4

OP:IP – outpatient:inpatient.

FURTHER READING

All social services including health

Family Welfare Association. *Guide to the Social Services*. London: Family Welfare Association, published annually.

Health services

Children

Acheson R. M., Hagard S. (1984) Services for children and physically and mentally handicapped. In: *Health, Society and Medicine: an Introduction to Community Medicine*, pp. 323–342. Oxford: Blackwell Scientific Publications

The elderly

Department of Health and Social Security (1978) *A Happier Old Age*. London: HMSO

Scottish Home and Health Department (1980) *Changing Patterns of Care*. Edinburgh: HMSO

Scottish Home and Health Department (1980) *The Elderly with Mental Illness*. Edinburgh: HMSO

Nursing

Henderson V. (1968) *Basic Principles of Nursing Care*. International Council of Nursing. Basle: Eskarger

Planning, direction

Department of Health and Social Security (1974) *Social Work Support for the Health Service*. London: HMSO (Evidence to working party)

Department of Health and Social Security (1976) *Priorities for Health and Social Services in England*. London: HMSO

Department of Health and Social Security (1976) *Sharing Resources for Health in England*. London: HMSO (Report of the resource allocation working party, RAWP)

Department of Health and Social Security (1977) *The Way Forward. Priorities in the Health and Social Services*. London: HMSO

Department of Health and Social Security (1981) *Care in Action – a Handbook of Policies and Priorities for the Health and Personal Social Services in England*. London: HMSO

Newell K. W. (1975) *Health by the People*. Geneva: World Health Organization

Roemer M. I., Roemer R. J. (1981) *Health Care Systems and Comparative Manpower Policies*. New York: Marcel Dekker Inc.

Scottish Home and Health Department (1976) *Health Services in Scotland. The Way Ahead*. Edinburgh: HMSO

Scottish Home and Health Department (1977) *Scottish Health Authorities Revenue Equalization* (SHARE). Edinburgh: HMSO

Scottish Home and Health Department (1980) *Scottish Health Authorities Priorities for the Eighties* (SHAPE). Edinburgh: HMSO

Process and outcome

Department of Health and Social Security (1980) *Inequalities in Health*. London: HMSO (Report of working group, chaired by Sir Douglas Black)

Department of Health and Social Security (1986) *Primary Health Care: an Agenda for Discussion*. London: HMSO

Kohn R., White K. L. (1976) *Health Care: an International Study*. Oxford: Oxford University Press

Royal Commission on the National Health Service (1979) *Report*. London: HMSO Cmnd 7615 (Chairman: Sir Alex Merrison)

Structure

Department of Health and Social Security (1984) *Implementation of the NHS Management Inquiry Report (Griffiths Report)*. London: HMSO

Levitt R. (1984) *Reorganised National Health Service*, p. 131. London: Croom Helm

Chapter
5

Health and Behaviour

**ILLNESS BEHAVIOUR ● DOCTOR–PATIENT RELATIONSHIP ●
DISTRIBUTION OF ILL-HEALTH IN THE UK**

This chapter deals with the patient's point of view and with concepts in society about what constitutes health and sickness. Even the most modern medical technology and the most efficient health service in the world will still have little effect on people's health or illness if they are not willing and able to use what is available. The most important determinant of health is people's behaviour – what they regard as illness, how they react to it, and how patients and health professions relate to each other.

As members of society, medical students already have personal knowledge of human behaviour and have concepts and experience of behaviour about health and illness. The purpose of medical training is to expand that knowledge to include the varying concepts and behaviour of the individuals who will, at some time, seek help and information from doctors, and of the doctors who provide such help.

Most doctors deal with a wide cross-section of society. The principles which shape behaviour in relation to health will act as a framework in which a patient can be better understood and the doctor–patient relationship and treatment can be adapted accordingly. They also form a basis for improving techniques of promotion and maintenance of health in people who are well.

A wider issue is the changes in population age-structure, in life styles and in patterns of disease and illness which were summarized in the Introduction and in Chapter 4. Such change is a continuous process in any open society and an understanding of how it arises and accumulates is essential if medicine as a whole is to be adaptable to the challenges which face it.

OBJECTIVES

Students should know:

(1) that definitions of normality in relation to health and illness vary in type (e.g. statistical or cultural, lay or professional)
(2) that an individual's recognition and management of illness is influenced both by social factors, which vary between cultures and groups in society and also by differences in the lay and medical care available
(3) the varying ways in which patients may move through the medical care system (e.g. from receptionist to general practitioner to nurse) and the factors which influence each decision to allocate clinical care
(4) the usual impact on families of someone being 'sick' and the ways in which this may affect the actions of doctors and other health professionals.

Students should be able to:

(1) apply simple methods of studying societies and groups
(2) define precisely the questions which any such study is intended to answer
(3) give several possible explanations for variations in patterns of illness or care
(4) list the problems in obtaining valid information by questionnaire
(5) recognize in an individual patient the factors which increase or decrease the amount of help sought and the likely extent of compliance with advice and instruction
(6) list the cultural and social factors which influence the relationship between doctor and patient
(7) apply probabilities in describing illness behaviour and medical care.

Students should appreciate:

(1) that the various health care professions inevitably have different priorities and values which may conflict with each other
(2) that cultural and social differences are just as important in health-promoting behaviour as in disease causation.

ILLNESS BEHAVIOUR

By illness behaviour we mean not simply how people react to feeling ill, but rather how symptoms are perceived and experienced, how they are interpreted, the actions that are taken and why, the factors that determine the decision to seek help and its timing. The relevance for doctors is that these considerations determine whether treatment commences at all, and influence whether or not the patient cooperates. If there are systematic differences between groups of the population, this has obvious implications at the widest level for health care systems and public health programmes. At the level of the doctor faced with an individual patient, the study of illness behaviour helps him to understand the patient's point of view and to provide a more effective service.

Disease, illness, sickness and fitness

First, it is useful, simply as an aid to conceptual clarity, to distinguish these terms.

Disease refers to abnormal physical or psychological processes, associated with characteristic sets of symptoms. In a classic paper, *Disease versus Illness in General Practice*, Helman (1981) defines it thus:

> 'Diseases are the named pathological entities that make up the medical model of ill-health, such as diabetes or tuberculosis, and which can be specifically identified and described by reference to certain biological, chemical or other evidence. In a sense, diseases are seen as abstract 'things' or independent entities which have specific properties and a recurring identity in whichever setting they appear. That is, they are assumed to be universal in their form, progress and content. Their aetiology, symptoms and signs, natural history, treatment and prognoses are considered to be similar in whatever individual, culture or group they occur. The universality of the form of a disease is related to the medical model's definitions of health and normality. In many cases, it is assumed that normality can be defined by reference to certain physical and biochemical parameters such as weight, height, haemoglobin level, blood counts, level of electrolytes or hormones, blood pressure, heart rate and so on. For each measurement there is a numerical range within which the individual is healthy and normal. Disease is often seen as a deviation from these normal values, and accompanied by abnormalities in the structure or function of body organs or systems. Aspects

of personality, such as intelligence, can also be quantified within a numerical range of normality, for instance in IQ tests'.

Illness, on the other hand, is a subjective state, the response of the individual to his or her perception of signs and symptoms. Disease may exist without illness, and illness may also exist without (identified) disease. Helman, again, points out that:

> 'the *disease model* assumes that diabetes in a Manchester patient is the same as diabetes in a New Guinea tribesman. While their blood glucose levels may be identical, the meaning of the disease to the patients, and the strategies they adopt to deal with it, may be very different in the two cases. The disease model cannot deal with such personal, cultural and social factors in ill-health, which are better viewed from the perspective of illness'.

Sickness is the term used for the role of the ill person; it refers to the expectations and obligations that society has of someone who is ill, and is, of course, even more dependent upon social norms than is 'illness'. If a condition is severe or incapacitating, the patient has no choice about adopting the role of one who is sick: he or she becomes dependent on others, retires to bed, and is unable to carry out the normal functions of everyday life. If there is any choice, however, there may be doubt about whether or not it is legitimate to take up a sick role. Should the patient 'give in' or struggle on? Would it be proper to stay away from work or not? Is this condition really an illness for which one might expect help and consideration from other people? The answers to such questions depend on the individual's social characteristics, his age, for instance, and also on the culture in which he lives. Ultimately, the doctor is the person who makes the sick role legitimate.

Fitness is a rather different concept, because it is concerned with more positive health, referring to a level of physiological or psychological functioning rather than simply to the absence or presence of disease or illness. An individual may be very fit (for his or her age) even though temporarily ill. Conversely, he may perceive himself as unfit, leading an unhealthy life and not at the peak of physical or mental condition, without any disease.

The illness 'career'

It is statistically normal to experience frequent signs or symptoms which could be defined as disease or illness. Large-scale surveys which ask respondents about the symptoms they have experienced during a defined period such as 2 weeks, usually find that up to 90% claim to have perceived one or more illness episodes. Obviously, not all these are taken for medical attention. Table 5.1 demonstrates the frequency of symptoms, and the action taken for them in one survey in London. It will be noted that lay action was, in fact, more common than medical treatment.

Table 5.1   *Random sample of 1000 adults resident in London. Incidence of symptoms, and action taken, over 14-day period*

Individuals with no symptoms	49
Individuals with symptoms, but no action taken	188
Individuals with symptoms, taking non-medical action	562
Individuals attending general practitioner	168
Individuals attending hospital outpatients	28
Individuals admitted as hospital inpatients	5
Total	1000

Adapted from Wadsworth *et al.*, 1971

The first stages of the illness 'career' are shown in Fig. 5.1. Some of the factors which may affect decisions at each stage are:

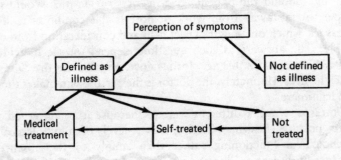

Figure 5.1   The illness 'career'.

First stage: the perception of symptoms

Perception of symptoms may depend on:

(1) characteristics of the individual, including his tolerance threshold and his state of stress or anxiety

(2) the concepts of normality held within a given social group, such as an age-group or an ethnic group

(3) the individual's own knowledge of his 'normal' state.

Second stage: the interpretation of symptoms

The meaning that is given to the symptom, whether or not it is defined as illness, may depend on:

(1) the nature and duration of the symptom

(2) its familiarity or novelty, in relation to an individual medical history

(3) the patient's knowledge of the meaning of symptoms, assumptions about the cause and prognosis of the disorder

(4) the possibility of normalization and rationalization — is there any 'obvious' explanation which means that the symptom need not be taken seriously?

Third stage: the decision whether to seek treatment

Whether or not medical advice is seen as appropriate may depend on:

(1) the extent to which the symptoms interfere, potentially or actually, with normal activities or with some important event

(2) the effect on other people around, and the amount of sympathy or sanctioning received, which may vary according to the visibility or functional consequences of the symptom

(3) the lay advice received from a particular network of friends and relations (and especially, in the case of married people, from a spouse)

(4) the costs and benefits of being defined as 'sick'

(5) barriers (practical or financial) to seeking medical care, the availability of medical services, and the experiences on which assumptions about approved consultation behaviour are based

(6) the success or otherwise of any attempt at self-treatment.

The pathway by which the patient reaches the consulting-room may thus be complicated. In the light of this, both the neglect of symptoms which should be treated and, on the other hand, a seeming over-readiness to consult for self-limiting conditions, can be better understood. Many research studies (such as that of Robinson, 1971) offer examples of the difficult decision-making that goes on within families, in the context of everyday worries and priorities. This suggests that it is important for the doctor to consider not only 'why has this patient come to consult about these symptoms?' but also 'why has he come now, at this particular moment?'

Lay concepts of health and illness

Behaviour can rarely be predicted from an individual's or a group's general attitudes to health, and generalizations are dangerous. As the above list of factors influencing the illness career has suggested, there are too many fortuitous and situational variables which may intervene. However, general orientations towards health and illness do differ between social and cultural groups, and may be important both for the understanding of the individual patient's behaviour and for the guidance of health education programmes.

Some basic themes are found in many different cultures. Even in educated and industrialized populations, a moral undertone still attaches to health and illness, although obviously not as strongly as in primitive cultures. Thus illness can be stigmatized, and be accompanied by feelings of guilt. Other themes commonly combine very fundamental notions with concepts learned from scientific medicine: the idea of a reserve of resistance is one, and the concept of susceptibility, of disease being ever-present and waiting for a trigger, is another. There is a general human need to explain, to connect together, for it is frightening to face a random world. One consequence of this is a common habit of giving more weight than medical science might allow to heredity and 'family failings'.

Other distinct concepts of health and illness are found among particular social groups. Ethnic groups, and older people in different geographical areas, may of course have specific cultural beliefs, often based on a long-term view of the group's medical history. Health may also have different meanings for the fortunate and for the socially deprived. Those who have done manual work all their lives may expect a quicker 'wearing out' of the body and accept lower standards of what it is to be normally healthy. Fitness has been found to be a less salient concept for people in poor circumstances. It is the better educated who are more likely to have a positive model of health as fitness, not simply the absence of illness, and so stress the importance of lifestyles and behavioural factors; the disadvantaged may well, with some logic, take a fatalistic view of health as outside their own control. This has implications for health education and preventive medicine.

In a sense, however, every family has its own health 'culture', based on accumulated experience and knowledge. It is not helpful to think of these lay models as being in opposition to medical models; rather, they should be respected as having their own logic and importance in influencing illness behaviour. As Helman (1981) concluded:

'The doctor's view of the disease process must be reconciled with the patient's subjective view of his own illness and contradictions between the two models must be resolved by the process of negotiation. Both the diagnosis and the prescribed treatment must make sense in terms of the patient's lay models of illness or they will not be accepted.'

DOCTOR–PATIENT RELATIONSHIPS

The ways in which doctor–patient relationships are structured and function are of considerable importance to the satisfactory practice of medicine. This is because illness and health are social, as well as medical, concepts. Amongst other things, this means that patients and doctors each bring to the surgery or consulting room expectations, rights, responsibilities and obligations, as well as background knowledge and experience, which structure the ways in which they relate to each other and thus affect the outcome of medical care.

Doctor, patient and society

As indicated in Fig. 5.2, the doctor enters his/her relationship not just as a private citizen, but as a member of the medical profession. This defines, and confines, his/her actions in a number of ways. For instance, there are standards of professional behaviour and ethics which determine what is acceptable medical practice. Thus, doctors are expected to treat all individuals objectively, regardless of race, colour, creed or sex. They are not allowed to exploit their privileged access to the human mind and body for personal or sexual gain. In addition, there are interprofessional relations within medicine which structure, for instance, the ways in which general practitioners and specialists relate to each other and to patients whom they see professionally. In Fig. 5.2, reference is made to 'subcultural reference groups' and these relate to factors such as class, race and religion which may play a part in a doctor's approach to his/her medical work and patients. One notable factor here is that the majority of doctors come from professional and middle-class backgrounds; from these they bring certain values, standards of behaviour and concepts of health and illness which may be different from those held by patients from other social and occupational backgrounds.

Patients also bring background experiences and influences from their own immediate environment and subcultural reference groups. The family is one major influence, especially with regard to what is

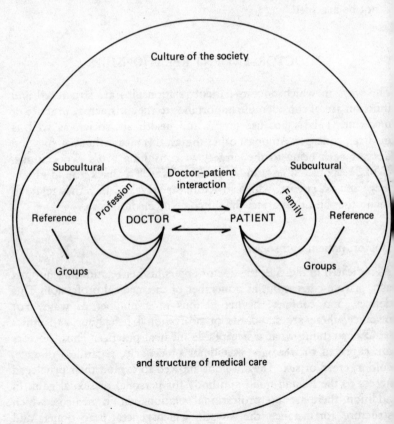

Figure 5.2   Doctor–patient interaction (adapted from Bloom, 1963).

defined as illness and what should be done about it. Other subcultural reference groups include work mates and colleagues, social friends, religious affiliations and ethnic groups.

The subcultural influences of both patients and doctors must also be located within the wider sociocultural context (*see* Fig. 5.2) of the society in which they live. Thus, in a country like the USA, where medical care is largely organized around the principles of the market economy, both patients' and doctors' expectations of medical practice may be quite different to those in a country such as the UK, where a national health service is dominant. (For more detailed comparisons of services *see* p. 121.)

Sources of potential conflict

The sociologist Freidson (1970) suggested that the worlds of professional doctors and lay patient 'are always in potential conflict with one another'. Some sources of this latent conflict are:

(1) There are many ways in which the patient's perception of his condition may differ from his doctor's. The patient may focus upon illness and the doctor on disease.

(2) Lay and professional viewpoints may clash, not only because each may bring different values from their own subcultures, as noted above, but also because each is specialized in a different way. The doctor's knowledge is that of the trained expert, the patient's is a subjective experience of his own body.

(3) Both may, however, be working in a context of uncertainty. The doctor knows that there are limitations within medical knowledge, and that each patient is an individual about whom perfect predictions can rarely be made. The patient's uncertainty derives from his relative medical ignorance. Both may find this uncertainty difficult to handle.

(4) Conflict is also inherent in the different saliences which the interaction may have for the two participants. The doctor sees many patients; the patient may consult only rarely.

(5) Increasingly, there may be conflict and uncertainty about what constitutes a 'proper' medical problem. Since doctors themselves vary in the extent to which they are interested in psychosocial problems, or see them as an appropriate task, there is potential for a considerable clash of expectations.

Communication

Various models of the doctor–patient relationship have been sugges-ted. A classic paper by Szasz and Hollender (1956), for instance, proposed three distinct types of relationship:

(1) activity–passivity, where the patient is totally passive (a model more appropriate to acute conditions or totally helpless states)
(2) guidance–cooperation, where the doctor advises and the patient cooperates (the most usual model)
(3) mutual participation, where the role of the doctor is to help the patient to manage his own condition (a model appropriate to long-term chronic conditions).

Obviously this is a very simple classification and many relationships change over time and even during a consultation. However, it does highlight the different roles that doctors have to be able to play.

The mode of interaction adopted obviously dictates the nature of the communication which develops between doctor and patient. Byrne and Long (1976) analysed 2500 interviews between patients of all social groups and general practitioners within the NHS, and found a continuum from a 'doctor-centred' style, with little participation by the patient except to answer questions, to a wholly 'patient-oriented' style, where the doctor spent much time listening and reflecting, as shown in Fig. 5.3. Most of the consultations analysed came into the 'doctor-oriented' categories.

In fact, in studies of patients' views of medical care, communication is always found to be the major source of any dissatisfaction. In particular, patients express special needs for the explanation and discussion which a busy doctor all too often cannot find time to give them:

'Suffering without explanation is particularly hard to bear. Thus the disturbing reality of disease experience gives rise to questions – why me? and why now? The offering of a diagnosis or label is not

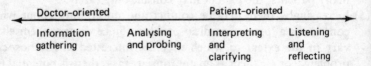

Figure 5.3 Mode of communication.

enough and anxiety will be alleviated only if some indication is given of how the situation might have come about.' (Wood and Bury, 1979).

A doctor who listens is the ideal expressed in many surveys of patients. If communication is felt to be inadequate, this has considerable consequences for patient behaviour and the response to advice.

Compliance

Communication must also be efficient. Ley and Spelman (1965) found in a series of studies in different settings that between one-third and one-half of the information given to patients was not recalled soon after the consultation. Patients were found to recall best what was heard first (which was more likely to refer to diagnosis rather than treatment). Even if advice is understood, however, compliance with it can never be assumed. Many studies have considered adherence to prescribed drugs regimens, finding considerable variations. Elderly people, in particular, may not take drugs as they are prescribed: the particularly detailed study by Wandless *et al.* (1979) of patients aged over 65 (by interviews, tablet counts at home, and examination of records) found that over half were taking considerably less, or more, than the prescribed dosage. The taking of drugs is, indeed, one area where the effect of conflicting expectations of the medical consultation can be clearly seen. Whereas doctors have frequently been found to say that patients too frequently expect drugs to be prescribed, on the other hand, all surveys of the public find that 'doctors are too ready to prescribe' is one of the most frequent complaints.

Similarly, non-compliance with advice is very frequently found in studies of antenatal care or dietary instructions. In acute and incapacitating illness, the patient has little choice about its management. In other circumstances, however, he or she will have a range of personal priorities and practical constraints to consider, and treatment may be perceived as having costs as well as benefits. Particularly in long-term or chronic illness, patients have to develop individual strategies for coping with their disease and maintaining normal life as far as possible.

Conclusion

Given the variability of patients' and doctors' background influences and experiences, variations in illness types and degrees of severity, and the existence of medical uncertainty, it becomes clear that it is unwise to talk about *the* doctor–patient relationship. There are many varieties of relationship, not only along these dimensions, but also in terms of conflict and consensus. That is to say, where doctors' and patients' background influences and experiences are similar, and where they share a common definition of the nature of the presenting condition and their respective roles in its management, and when medical uncertainty is low, one would anticipate a generally smooth and conflict-free relationship between doctor and patient. Where any, or all, of these factors fail to hold, there is potential for conflict. Conflict, however, is not necessarily a bad thing; it may lead to discussion and better understanding, and its careful management by both doctors and patients can lead to satisfactory resolution, contributing to more effective medical care.

THE DISTRIBUTION OF ILL-HEALTH IN THE UK

Figures 5.4 and 5.5 and Tables 5.2 and 5.3 show some examples of the way in which rates of ill health vary in the UK by broad factors such as age, sex, geographical area and social class.

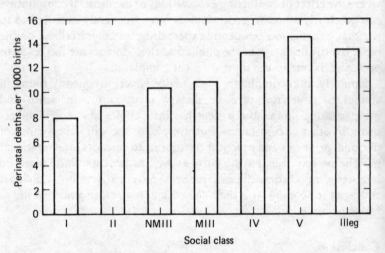

Figure 5.4 Perinatal mortality by legitimacy and social class of father in England and Wales (source OPCS Monitor DH3 84.6).

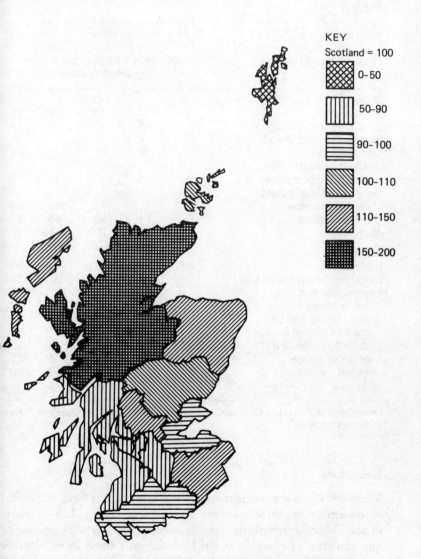

Figure 5.5 Standardized mortality ratios for road traffic accidents in Scotland (Registrar General's Report, 1982, by Health Board Area of Residence).

Table 5.2 *Chronic sickness: prevalence of reported limiting long-standing illness by sex, age, and socio-economic group (All persons, Great Britain: 1982)*

Age (years) Socio-economic group	0–15	16–44	45–64	65 and over	Total
	Percentage who reported limiting long-standing illness				
Males					
Professional	8	7	17	[14]	11
Employers and managers	5	10	17	37	14
Intermediate and junior non-manual	6	8	26	42	15
Skilled manual and own account non-professional	7	10	27	41	17
Semi-skilled manual and personal service	4	12	31	47	20
Unskilled manual	3	12	38	40	23
All males	6	10	26	41	17
Females					
Professional	3	10	14	[13]	10
Employers and managers	4	9	21	37	14
Intermediate and junior non-manual	6	11	23	40	17
Skilled manual and own account non-professional	5	13	26	45	18
Semi-skilled manual and personal service	5	14	32	48	25
Unskilled manual	7	13	33	50	30
All females	5	12	26	45	19

From Office of Population Censuses and Surveys (1984) *General Household Survey, 1982* London: HMSO.

Definitions

These variations are considerable. In trying to explain them, it is useful to remember the three concepts distinguished on pp. 128–9. Some of the Tables clearly show rates of *disease* (e.g. mortality figures, or any statistics of clinically-defined conditions); some show rates of *illness*, (e.g. people reporting themselves as ill, or people consulting a general practitioner); and some show rates of *sickness* (e.g. people whose activity is restricted, or who are away from work). The way in

Table 5.3 *Standardized mortality ratios[1] based on UK experience (UK = 100), 1983, males and females*

Cause (ICD codes)[1]	Scotland M	Scotland F	England M	England F	Wales M	Wales F	Northern Ireland M	Northern Ireland F
All causes	117	119	97	97	116	107	97	93
Cancers and other neoplasms	109	117	99	99	100	102	66	72
Myocardial infarction and other ischaemic heart disease	125	123	95	97	126	109	114	107
Strokes and other cerebrovascular disease	155	153	94	93	119	119	109	122
Chronic bronchitis ephysema and asthma	55	60	104	105	157	95	49	50
All accidents, poisonings and violence	197	238	86	85	84	115	270	146

[1] See Chapter 2.
Source: Adapted from Table 2.14, *Regional Trends – 1985* Central Statistical Office, HMSO 1985.

which the statistics are constructed – medical records, self-reports, administrative records – obviously depends on the aspect of 'ill-health' being considered.

Possible explanations

In understanding patterns of ill-health among the population there are many different *modes of explanation* likely to be relevant. They may be difficult to disentangle, but it is important to consider all of them when creating hypotheses for further exploration.

(1) Biological variables: age, sex and ethnic group are obviously biological (although they also have social meanings).
(2) Environmental variables: some of the differences between geographical areas, or between rural/urban areas, or between social classes, are due to factors in the external environment – climate, pollution, agents in working environments.

(3) Life-style and behaviour variables: behaviours such as smoking, alcohol consumption, eating habits, are clearly relevant, as is the general environment of poverty.
(4) Factors concerned with the perception and definition of illness: different standards will obviously apply to babies, young men, the elderly, and different meanings will be given to their symptoms.
(5) Factors which determine the individual's decision to seek help: these create rates of consultation, and so may affect rates of referral to and use of various services.
(6) Variables of health-service provision: many statistics are rates of provision, rather than rates of need (*see* Chapter 4).

The simple variables which can demonstrate 'inequality' in health chances among the population may combine the effects of several of these in a complicated manner. There are always differences, for instance, by marital status, with the single (at older ages) and the divorced or separated showing higher mortality rates and poorer health than the married, especially among men. It may be that married men have more favourable environments and lifestyles. The effect of selection must also be considered, however, perhaps the unmarried or the divorced include some of the least healthy groups.

Similarly, data about geographical differences in mortality are reasonably reliable and, as can be seen in Table 5.3, give rise to concern and enquiry about why there is still wide variation throughout such a supposedly homogeneous population as the UK. But, in examining these differences, many modes of possible explanation have to be considered. Biological factors of the genetic make-up of populations may be relevant. The physical environment – climate, water hardness, pollution – may be important. The social environment, including the relative prosperity of different regions, must be taken into account, as must behavioural factors such as typical diets, or levels of smoking and alcohol consumption. The occupational structure of areas differs, and so do the numbers of the unemployed or the retired. Finally, the standard of available services may vary: this is unlikely to have a great effect upon health statistics (and indeed better services may apparently *increase* some statistics of ill-health), but may be a factor for some groups of the population in particularly disadvantaged areas such as inner cities.

Again, there may be important differences between the health of ethnic minorities and the native population because of biological variables relating to susceptibility to specific diseases. But the social environment typical of different groups – their occupations, poverty or wealth, and geographical clustering – may be of greater overall importance.

The Tables show that, at this nationwide level, great inequalities are still demonstrated by 'social class'. This is the clearest way in which health experience differs in the population, and a fact which gives rise to much concern. How is it that, after nearly 40 years or so of a freely available health service, these variations do not seem to have been greatly diminished? But 'social class' is also one of the most complex variables, involving all the modes of explanation listed above.

It was in the mid-nineteenth century that striking differences in mortality between different occupations was first noted in Britain. These might partly be explained by the specific hazards of different types of work, but it seemed probable that the social environment of poverty, poor nutrition, housing, exposure to infection and poor medical care, was also important. The early social surveys of the pioneers, such as Booth in London or Rowntree in York, pointed to the need for social classifications in attempts to examine the difference between the health of the poor and the rich. Thus, since 1911, mortality statistics have been provided by the Registrar General's social class, and many other health data are analysed by this and other classifications.

The Registrar General's classification of occupation (social class)

It is important to be clear that the basic Registrar General's social classes I–V is an *occupational* classification. Families are classified according to the occupation of the 'head of the household'. Crudely, the six social classes are defined as follows:

I   professional occupations
II   managerial and senior administrative occupations
IIIN non-manual occupations such as clerical workers or shop assistants
IIIM skilled manual occupations
IV   semi-skilled manual occupations
V   unskilled occupations

Classes I–IIIN are sometimes called 'non-manual classes' and IIIM–V 'manual classes'. The terms 'middle' or 'working' class should be avoided, as they have no precise meaning. It must be noted that social class IIIM is by far the largest in the (male) population, almost 40% of the whole. Classes I and V are both relatively small. Non-manual males comprise about one-third of the male population, and manual two-thirds.

Although this classification has the advantage of continuity of use over so many years, and demonstrates its usefulness by the clarity and regularity of the patterns which are produced, it has some obvious problems.

(1) The nature or the importance of a particular occupation changes over time. In the smaller population of 1911 there were a million agricultural labourers and nearly 400 000 male domestic servants in social class V in England and Wales, both are now smaller proportions of the population, and are graded in social class IV. Up until 1931, male clerks were assigned to social class II, but the spread of education meant some loss of status for this occupational group and it is now classified as IIIN.

(2) For mortality figures, occupation is taken as that which is recorded on death certificates. This may be unclear, or not in fact the occupation followed for most of the individual's life.

(3) The classification does not distinguish between employers, the self-employed and employees.

(4) The earlier analyses of the mortality of married women were based solely on the occupation of their husbands. Increasingly, however, alternative methods are being used: classification by husband's occupation focuses on the socio-economic dimension of their lives, but additional analyses for the occupationally active wives draw attention to the fact that their own occupations may also be associated with their health. Single, divorced and widowed women have always been classified by their own occupation.

(5) There are clear associations between age and social mobility. In some occupations, status (and income) is likely to rise throughout life; in others, to fall towards the end of a working career. Health itself is an important influence both on initial selection into jobs and on mobility from one type of occupation to another. Thus occupation recorded at death may confuse these processes, and health status at any given age may be either the cause or the effect of occupational status.

In an attempt to provide alternative methods for dealing with these difficulties, many systems of social class categorization have been used and, in attempting to understand health statistics or generate from them hypotheses about the distribution of ill-health, it is important to note which classification is being employed. Alternatives to Registrar General social class include:

(1) *Occupation orders*, which describe the type of occupation or industry in which the individual works, rather than his status. There are 350 occupation units, combined into 17 occupation orders. Obviously these reflect more directly any specific hazards which are associated with work or its environment.

(2) The *socio-economic groups* (SEG) classification, which was introduced into official statistics in 1947, in an attempt to permit distinction between, for instance, professional employees and the self-employed and produce categories which as far as possible contained 'people whose social, cultural and recreational standards and behaviour are similar'. There are 16 socio-economic groups, sometimes compressed (as in the figures from the continuing national interview survey, the General Household Survey) into groups 1–6.

(3) *Market research* classifications, which are similar to but not identical with the Registrar General's social class. These are designated A, B, C1, C2 and D. Many of the occupations assigned to social class IV are here included in class C1.

(4) Several *sociological classifications* have been developed in an attempt to distinguish life-styles and life chances more clearly, or take into account the education or occupation of the mother as well as the father of a family. These, while they are not used in official statistics, may well be found in accounts of research. Examples are the Hope-Goldthorpe index, or the social index of the longitudinal birth cohort survey called 'Child Health and Education'.

(5) *The Office of Population Censuses and Surveys 1% longitudinal study*, while it uses the conventional social classes and socio-economic groups, represents an important development in overcoming the problems listed earlier. Beginning in the early 1970s, for a continuous 1% sample of the population, mortality, birth and other records are being related to the succeeding census records of the same individuals. This obviously offers great advantages over the conventional method of relating mortality simply to the 'pool' of the general population. Occupation and

socio-economic circumstances throughout life can, eventually, be related to mortality. Early analyses from this series have added considerably to knowledge about the distribution of that aspect of ill-health which is represented by mortality rates. It has been shown, for instance, that those who were unemployed, but seeking work at census in 1971 were more likely to die by 1975 than those who were employed. The complex association of social class with health disadvantage is illuminated, at this national level, by the demonstration that those without basic household amenities have greatly elevated mortality rates.

Whatever system is used, social class groupings are a complex classification, and statistics serve only as crude indicators of problems which need further investigation before anything can be said about causes. This is true also of regional differences, with which social class may be associated because of occupational patterns and levels of economic prosperity. For instance, the knowledge that in the UK there are class differences in perinatal mortality (*see* Fig. 5.4) requires the investigation of possible differences in underlying environmental, social, genetic and service provision factors. What might explain the fact that people in the same occupational class are not equally healthy, judged by mortality rates or the prevalence of illness, in south-east England, in the Midlands, and in Scotland? What possible explanations might there be for the fact that there is always a marked social class difference in reported chronic or long-standing illness, but little in acute illness?

The methods of investigating these questions are described in Chapter 2. Always, of course, one is dealing with *probabilities* and groups, and saying nothing about the health of the individual. But, at both the population and the individual level, it is essential to look clearly, first, at the nature of the evidence. Then, it is necessary to consider several sorts of evidence together, and to break out of accustomed moulds of thinking in terms of only one type of explanation. This applies to an overemphasis upon the psychological, reducing all ailments to the psychosomatic, as much as to an exclusive focus upon the biological. All modes of explanation have to be taken together, not forgetting the social, the behavioural, the environmental and the boundaries set by systems of medical care. The aim is to indicate the most effective action in terms of both prevention and treatment.

REFERENCES AND FURTHER READING

This Study Guide contains references specific to topics as they arise, but there are a few texts which are worthwhile as additional reading.

General

Armstrong D. (1983) *An Outline of Sociology as Applied to Medicine.* Bristol: Wright & Sons

Robinson D. (1978) *Patients, Practitioners and Medical Care.* London: Heinemann Medical

Tuckett D. (1976) *An Introduction to Medical Sociology.* London: Tavistock

Illness behaviour

Blaxter M., Paterson E. (1982) *Mothers and Daughters: Health Attitudes and Behaviour in Two Generations.* London: Heinemann Educational

Eisenberg L. (1977) Disease and illness: distinctions between professional and popular ideas of sickness. *Culture, Medicine and Psychiatry,* 1: 9–23

Helman C. G. (1981) Disease versus illness in general practice. *Journal of the Royal College of General Practitioners* 31: 230, 548–52

Pill R., Stott N. C. H. (1982) Concepts of illness causation and responsibility: some preliminary data from a sample of working class mothers. *Social Science and Medicine,* 16: 43–52

Robinson D. (1971) *The Process of Becoming Ill.* London: Routledge & Kegan Paul

Wadsworth M. E. J. (1971) Butterfield W. J. H., Blaney R. (1971) *Health and Sickness: the Choice of Treatment.* London: Tavistock

Doctor–patient relationships

Bloom S. W. (1963) *The Doctor and his Patient,* p. 236. New York: Russell Sage Foundation

Byrne P., Long E. (1976) *Doctors Talking to Patients.* London: HMSO

Cartwright A., Anderson R. (1981) *General Practice Revisited: a Second Study of Patients and their Doctors.* London: Tavistock

Dunnell K., Cartwright A. (1972) *Medicine Takers, Prescribers and Hoarders.* London: Routledge & Kegan Paul

Freidson E. (1970) *Profession of Medicine.* New York: Dodd Mead

Ley P., Spelman M. S. (1965) Communications in an outgoing patient setting. *British Journal of Social and Clinical Psychology*, **4**: 114

Szasz T., Hollender M. (1956) The basic models of the doctor–patient relationship. *Archives of Internal Medicine*, **97**: 588

Wandless I., Mucklow J. C., Smith A., Prudham D. (1979) Compliance with prescribed medicines; a study of elderly patients in the community. *Journal of the Royal College of General Practitioners*, **29**: 391–6

Wood P. H. N., Bury M. R. (1979) Communication in chronic illness. *International Rehabilitation Medicine*, **1**: 3

Examples of studies

Cox C., Mead A., eds (1975) *A Sociology of Medical Practice*. West Drayton: Collier-Macmillan

Acheson R. M., Aird L., eds (1976) *Seminars in Community Medicine*. Oxford: Oxford University Press, vol 1

Distribution of ill-health in the UK

Carter C. O., Peal J. (1976) *Equalities and Inequalities in Health*. London: Academic Press

Fox A. J., Goldblatt P. O. (1982) *Longitudinal Study: Sociodemographic Mortality Differentials*. London: Office of Population Censuses and Surveys, HMSO

Gray A. (1981) *On the Black Report: Inequalities in Health, a Summary and Comment*. Aberdeen: Health Economics Research Unit

Morris J. N. (1979) Social inequalities undiminished. *Lancet* i: 87

Office of Population Censuses and Surveys (1984) *General Households Survey 1982*. London: HMSO

Priorities for the Future

CLINICAL ADVANCES • COMMUNICATIONS TECHNOLOGY • PATIENT MANAGEMENT • MULTIPLE PROFESSIONS • PREVENTION • SELF-CARE • HEALTH FOR ALL 2000 • COMMUNITY MEDICINE

CLINICAL ADVANCES

Priorities for the future of community medicine are derived from the shape of health and medical care and the challenges facing them. Medical care cannot and should not be static and throughout the Study Guide several developments have been mentioned which have altered medical care in the past decade. They, and perhaps other unforeseen factors, will almost certainly continue to influence the way in which medicine is practised and to have implications for the daily work of both clinicians and community physicians.

There are continuing advances in clinical treatments. The main ones have been classified by Sir Douglas Black (1979):

(1) advances of a modest cost which can prevent or cure diseases (such as immunization, antenatal care and antibiotics)

(2) advances now involving a modest cost which do not cure but allow personal health efficiency to be maintained (such as monthly vitamin B_{12} for pernicious anaemia, replacement hormones and control of hypertension)

(3) advances which offer to preserve a reasonable level of health but which have a high cost (such as organ transplantation).

The speed at which the third group will continue to develop depends on the availability of resources and the assessment of net benefits. Techniques in this group have become matters of public debate on grounds of cost and ethics but they are the growing edge of twentieth century medicine and could in due course move into Black's category (2). While it is possible that surgical interventions, such as coronary artery surgery or implantation of artificial organs, might in future form a substantial part of doctors' work for patients of all ages, to date the growth of new techniques has been greater in biochemical interventions such as hormone replacement or chemical oncology. Recent advances such as the pharmacological treatment of peptic ulcer support the view that this approach will, in future, offer more refined therapies for chronic disease than will surgery (whether they will have fewer side-effects remains to be seen).

COMMUNICATIONS TECHNOLOGY

Automation and communications technology have also markedly affected patient management, again in the direction of allowing the recording and sharing of information without the patient necessarily having to contact various doctors. Biological monitors for use by patients and automated review of patients with chronic conditions, such as thyroid dysfunction, are but two examples. The use of computers for assisting clinical decision-making, for history-taking and for teaching appears to be both efficient and effective by aiding recall of information (de Dombal, 1979). Applications of computing in primary care are currently being promoted by central government and could increase efficiency as well as quality of care.

'Distance-diagnosis', such as transmission of ECGs by telephone or the use of two-way telephone or visual display units, has been developed for rural areas and could be of value in providing health care for inner cities or poorly-staffed districts. In the relatively near future, digital technology may make possible a radiology department without x-ray films, although the cost may be prohibitive for some years to come. All of these developments increase the opportunities to decentralize care away from hospitals and from major centres of population. Expert domiciliary care is now feasible, although whether it is acceptable is a different question.

PATIENT MANAGEMENT

Patient management has also altered, mainly in the direction of reducing length of hospitalization. Day surgery, possible in part because of improvements in anaesthesia, has increased and there is scope for its further growth with the use of new technologies such as lasers. The 'sharing' or integration of care by specialists and general practitioners, whereby they follow an agreed management plan regardless of where and by whom the patient is seen, is being developed as a means of avoiding recurring visits to hospital. It has become possible in part because increased knowledge of risk factors, derived from epidemiological studies, allows the determination of more precise guidelines. The professional development of general practice has undoubtedly also contributed, as has the government's policy of reducing the numbers of acute hospital beds. Common examples are shared obstetric care and monitoring of long-term problems such as hypertension, all of which have arisen because of greater precision in defining risk or precursors of problems. There is, however, still much research to be done before we understand and can quantify risk for many major medical conditions so that intervention can be finely tuned to reduce overmedication and unnecessary side-effects.

MULTIPLE PROFESSIONS

Another trend has been the steady increase in the numbers of health professions allied to medicine. The greatest growth has been in scientific staff (*see* Table 4.1), laboratory scientists and clinical psychologists, with physical therapists, pharmacists and opticians not far behind. Nurses have taken on a widening range of tasks and special interests. This is most obvious in primary care, where the bulk of the enormous increase in caring for older, dependent patients has been met by district nurses. The current debate about teamwork in primary health care revolves in part around giving nurses greater professional autonomy and could result in important changes in the pattern of medical work in the UK. Certainly, the days of the isolated medical practitioner are past, nevertheless a proportion, albeit decreasing, of general practitioners still works single-handed. An important effect of this is the much greater need for organization and coordination within every patient-care setting, so that patients are not confused by a multiplicity of conflicting advice and treatment.

PREVENTION

More speculative is the future shape of preventive medicine within the

NHS. Although there are moves to increase the extent of screening and specific primary preventive techniques, such as immunization, which are carried out by primary health care teams, there are signs of a growing split between these and the more diffuse forms of prevention, namely health promotion by education and regulation. Most professions now attempt 'patient education' of ill patients as part of treatment, but primary health education, although increasingly sought by the public in the search for long-term health, is currently sitting uneasily within the health service. There is a growing acceptance of the fact that the single most important factor which would prevent disease and illness in those who suffer most is the reduction of poverty (DHSS, 1980), a strategy to which health services can contribute little other than by being more accessible. Thus it could be that the role of doctors in promoting health and preventing disease may increasingly become that of expert witnesses about cause and effect rather than as primary practitioners. Instead, the initiative for health promotion and education will come from politicians and communities, through public action such as reducing environmental stress factors and open debate about what constitutes a healthy life-style. Those in the health professions will be equal but not leading contributors to the search for health and will act mainly as a source of expert information.

It seems likely that secondary prevention by screening will concentrate more on physical disease with identifiable biological markers than on the more subjective variables of current programmes in child development and dependency in old age. As general health and fitness improve, the yield of unreported problems in both these age groups appears already to be falling, making them of dubious value. On the other hand, as more is learned about early biological changes in major diseases such as cancer, the opportunities for useful disease-screening programmes increase. However, it remains true that secondary prevention is usually a poor alternative to primary prevention if that can be achieved, even if only some of the risk factors for a multifactorial problem can be removed.

SELF-CARE

The growing trend towards greater personal responsibility for health is seen in the management of illness and the shape of medical care as well as in the prevention of disease. This trend has arisen for several reasons. The first and main one is the concept of self-determination, promoted worldwide since 1948 as a human right, which seeks greater individual autonomy in all aspects of living. Other factors are a growing concern about iatrogenic disease and a wish to be able to refuse major medical interventions; increased expectations of quick relief from minor illness for which Western medical care has no real answer; and the growing numbers of survivors who have to balance long-term management of chronic disease with leading a normal life. Thus one certain development for the future is a greater demand for doctors to explain, educate and negotiate with their patients over the management of illness. Although there is as yet no law of informed consent in the UK, recent judgements in medical law-suits reflect a belief in the public's right to know and to choose.

HEALTH FOR ALL 2000

The twin themes of the search for health and of lay participation in health care underlie what is potentially a major influence on the future work of community medicine, namely, the World Health Organization's policy *Targets for Health For All 2000* (1985) to which all nations are officially committed. It has three main elements: the promotion and facilitation of healthy lifestyles; a reduction in preventable ill-health; and a reorientation of health care systems towards primary health care. The strategy for all nations is to pursue the addition of years to life, of health to life, of life to years and equity in health. Thus in Europe, 38 targets for 2000 have been set which range from reducing by 25% the differences in health status between nations to increasing by 10% the average life span free from major disease and disability.

COMMUNITY MEDICINE

What do these trends imply for the future priorities of community medicine? The work of community medicine is derived from its particular blend of knowledge of social biology, clinical medicine and systems management. Community physicians are agents of change, helping to move health care towards the changing needs of communities as reflected in their mortality, local variations in disease patterns, and overall health, however measured.

In the 1974 health service reorganization in the UK, community medicine moved away from public health and towards health service management. This move was in line with the dominance at that time of hospital services over primary care. As a result, the focus for prevention within health services was lost. Now there is an opportunity and, indeed, pressure to restore both primary care and prevention to the forefront of attention. Public health is back in fashion.

At the same time, medical involvement in the management structure of the NHS has recently become less both for clinicians and for community physicians, as professional managers have taken on the new role of chief executive to a health authority. Community medicine is thereby freer to speak out again on behalf of health rather than of health authorities. In line with this re-emphasis of an old role, the Faculty of Community Medicine (1986) has adopted a set of targets for 2000 drawn from those of the European region; these require an active programme which involves many agencies outside the health service including schools, industry, the media and local government. Recently, a medical student expressed surprise at the amount of talking that went on in a doctor–patient consultation, but that indeed is the growing pattern of medical work both with patients and with public groups. Education and communication are the tools of health promotion.

The need for doctors trained in systems management remains. Of special importance is the development of coordinated community health care, probably built around the core primary care teams of general practitioners and community nurses. Neighbourhoods with high proportions of multiply deprived families require new strategies of domiciliary and community service delivery which cross practice boundaries, and local departments of community medicine must develop effective policies based on local epidemiology and knowledge of the community's own strengths and weaknesses. Another aspect of systems management is the development of communications networks which allow reliable and confidential transfer of patient information between different locations, and especially between home and hospital, without requiring the patient to move from one to the other for investigation or monitoring. Such systems must be based on an understanding of clinical needs, priorities and opportunities.

Finally, there has never been a greater need for community medicine's special concern with outcomes of care and monitoring of health status. The drive for greater efficiency in public services is unlikely to be reversed and is universal. The danger is that it concentrates attention on the use of resources rather than on what they achieve. Thus a fundamental and continuing task for community medicine is to apply epidemiology to producing useful measures of outcome for the evaluation and management of health services. The context of epidemiology may change but it will remain the basis of all population medicine and medical care.

REFERENCES

Black D. (1979) The paradox of medical care. *Journal of the Royal College of Physicians*, 13: 57–65

Department of Health and Social Security (1980) *Inequalities in Health*. Report of a working group chaired by Sir Douglas Black. London: HMSO

de Dombal, F. T. (1979) Picking the best test in acute abdominal pain. *Journal of the Royal College of Physicians* 13: 203–208

Faculty of Community Medicine of the Royal College of Physicians (1986) *Health for All 2000: Charter for Action*. London: FCM

World Health Organization Regional Office for Europe (1985) *Targets for Health for All 2000*. Copenhagen: WHO

Index